DENTAL ANATOMY AND ORAL HISTOLOGY

Simplified

(SCORE ORIENTED PERSPECTIVE)

Dr. Ravikumar S. Kulkarni.

Forwarded by

**Dr. Prabha Mallikarjun
Member of Parliament
Loksabha, Davangere,
Karnataka**

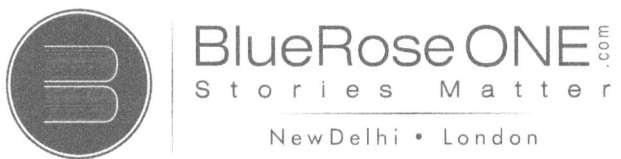

BLUEROSE PUBLISHERS
India | U.K.

Copyright © Dr. Ravikumar S. Kulkarni 2025

All rights reserved by author. No part of this publication may be reproduced, stored in a retrieval system or transmitted in any form or by any means, electronic, mechanical, photocopying, recording or otherwise, without the prior permission of the author. Although every precaution has been taken to verify the accuracy of the information contained herein, the publisher assumes no responsibility for any errors or omissions. No liability is assumed for damages that may result from the use of information contained within.

BlueRose Publishers takes no responsibility for any damages, losses, or liabilities that may arise from the use or misuse of the information, products, or services provided in this publication.

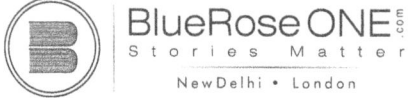

For permissions requests or inquiries regarding this publication,
please contact:

BLUEROSE PUBLISHERS
www.BlueRoseONE.com
info@bluerosepublishers.com
+91 8882 898 898
+4407342408967

ISBN: 978-93-7018-098-7

Cover design: Yash Singhal
Typesetting: Namrata Saini

First Edition: May 2025

About the Author

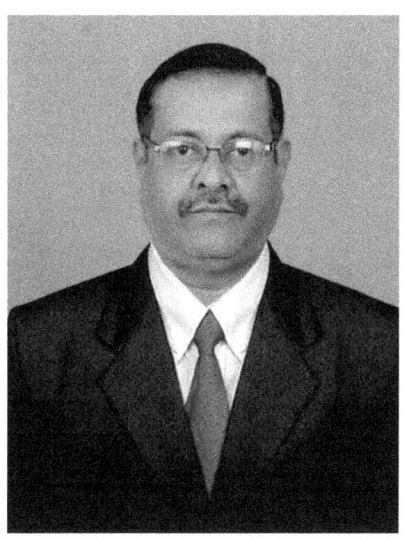

Author Dr. Ravikumar S. Kulkarni has done His BDS and MDS (Oral Pathology and Microbiology) from College of Dental Sciences, Davangere, Karnataka. He is currently working as Professor and Head in the Department of Oral Pathology and Microbiology, Daswani Dental College and Research Centre, Kota, Rajasthan. He has a vast 16 years of teaching experience for undergraduate, post-graduate and PhD students. He has numerous articles in his name published in both national and international journals. He has worked in various dental colleges across India.

About the Book

The book contains 15 years solved question papers taken from various Universities across India. As the book is oriented on exam based perspective, it is in question-answer pattern format. Questions are answered in a very simplified manner with illustrations which makes it easy for the students to understand and memorize.

The book is not only helpful for first year dental students; it can be helpful for interns preparing for NEET exam, Post-graduate students, nursing, dental hygienist, medical and pharmacy students.

Acknowledgement

I would like to express my deepest gratitude to all those who stood beside me to successfully complete this task.

I extend my sincere thanks to my mentor **Dr. Ram Manohar**, former Professor and Head, Department of Oral Pathology & Microbiology, College of Dental Sciences, Davangere, Karnataka, **Dr. Sunil S**, Vice Principal, Pushpagiri College of Dental Sciences, Tiruvalla, Kerala and **Dr. Madhushankari G.S**, Professor and Head, Department of Oral Pathology & Microbiology, College of Dental Sciences, Davangere, Karnataka for their invaluable guidance, constant support and feedback. Their experience and expertise in the field was helpful in writing the book.

I am also thankful to **Dr. Anil Daswani, Dr. Kanta Daswani** and **Er. Vijay Daswani** for providing necessary resources and infrastructure to carry out this work.

Special thanks to my colleagues, Staff members and students of Daswani Dental College and Research Centre, Kota, Rajasthan for their moral support.

Lastly, I am deeply grateful to my wife **Dr. Deeparani Horadi** and my children **Ruchi** and **Abhi** for their support and encouragement throughout this process.

Thank you all.

Dr. Ravikumar S. Kulkarni

DEDICATED IN LOVING MEMORY OF MY PARENTS

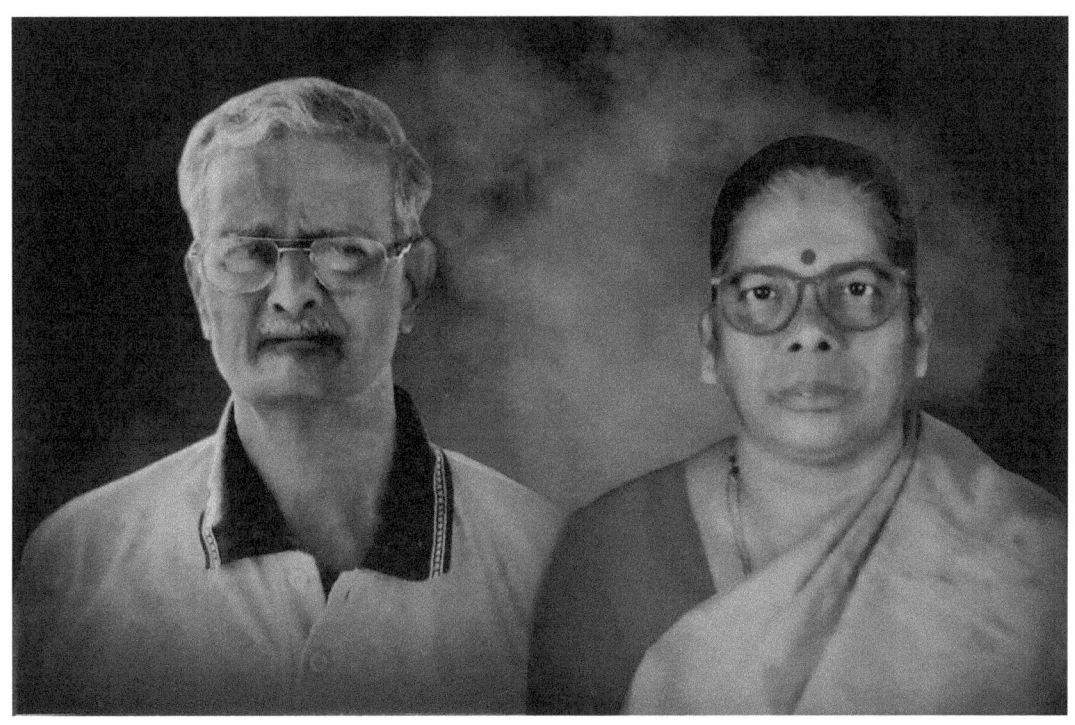

Late Shri Shivappa N. Kulkarni

Late Smt. Shaila S. Kulkarni

Preface

Writing this book was a challenging task and took me few years to complete. Understanding the basics of dentistry is fundamental not only for dental professionals but also for researchers and students. This book **[Dental Anatomy and Oral Histology – Simplified (Score oriented perspective)]** serves as a simple guide to Dental anatomy and Oral Histology. Years of study, teaching and experience in the field has resulted in this book. It is designed to simplify complex topics with clear explanations and diagrams that enhance better understanding of the subject. I have done my best to present it in a simple straight forward way. I hope this book will serve as a valuable tool.

I am greatful to all the people who supported me during this journey. I thank my family, colleagues and students who encouraged me in taking up this task.

Dr. Ravikumar S. Kulkarni
Professor & Head,
Department of Oral Pathology & Microbiology,
Daswani Dental College & Research Centre,
Kota - 325003,
Rajasthan

Tips How to Score in Exam

1) Attempt all questions.

2) Write answers in points so that it will be easy for the evaluators to correct.

3) Draw and label neat diagrams wherever necessary.

4) Write minimum 15 points for main question of ten marks and 8 points for short notes of five marks along with diagram.

5) Give first preference to important points of the question asked.

Dr. Ravikumar S. Kulkarni

Foreword

Understanding the complex structures and processes that control the health of our teeth and oral tissues is based on dental anatomy and oral histology. To properly diagnose, treat, and prevent oral illnesses, future dental practitioners must possess a thorough understanding of these topics. However, because of the intricacy and level of detail needed, studying dental anatomy and histology can frequently appear daunting, despite its significance.

This book "Dental Anatomy and Oral histology –Simplified" by Dr Ravikumar S Kulkarni, attempts to close that gap by making learning more engaging and approachable through its question-and-answer structure. In addition to simplifying the enormous amount of information, it promotes critical thinking and active participation by presenting questions and offering succinct, understandable responses. Whether you're a dental student preparing for exams, a practitioner revisiting fundamental concepts, or someone with a keen interest in understanding the detailed structure of the human mouth, this resource is designed to guide you through the essential topics with clarity and precision. The approach used here is designed to facilitate better retention, as it moves beyond rote memorization and helps you understand the logic behind the facts. This simplified version of Dental anatomy and Oral histology will help in easy understanding for health science students other than BDS too.

I hope that this book will be a useful guide for you as you explore the intriguing fields of oral histology and dental anatomy. May it not only contribute to your academic success but also inspire a lifelong passion for dentistry. To all dentists and medical professionals, let us serve society wherever and whenever it is needed, upholding the true spirit of healthcare.

Dr.Prabha Mallikarjun

Member of Parliament, Lok Sabha,
Davangere Constituency
Governing Council Member, BEA
SS Care Trust, Life Trustee

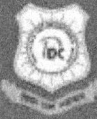

DASWANI DENTAL COLLEGE & RESEARCH CENTRE

Unit of : Aadarsh Pragya Vidhya Mandir Samiti

19-IPB, Institutional Area, RIICO, Ranpur, Kota - 325003 (Raj.)

Reg. No. 1/KOTA/1998-99 Dt. 3-4-1999
Fax : 0744-2505467

Ref. DDC/Acad/2667
Date 21/02/2025

Dear Dr. Ravikumar Kulkarni,

Heartfelt Congratulations on Your Book Release

It is with great pleasure that I extend my heartfelt congratulations to you on the release of your book. Your dedication and expertise in the field of Oral and Maxillofacial Pathology have always been commendable, and this remarkable achievement is a testament to your hard work and commitment to academic excellence.

Your contribution to dental education and research continues to inspire both students and colleagues alike. I am confident that your book will serve as a valuable resource for aspiring professionals in the field.

Wishing you continued success in all your future endeavours.

Warm regards,

Dr. Anil Daswani

Director,

Daswani Dental College & Research Centre, Kota

Foreword

It is with great pleasure that I write the foreword for the book titled Dental Anatomy and Oral Histology – Simplified (Score oriented prespective) authored by Dr. Ravikumar S Kulkarni, Professor & Head, Department of Oral Pathology & Microbiology, Daswani Dental College & Research Center, Kotta, Rajasthan, affiliated to Rajasthan University of Health Sciences, Jaipur, India

I am sure his wide range of academic capabilities and experience has helped him to compile this text book which covers the entire topics of Dental Anatomy & Oral histology in Question Answer format. This book shall cater to the needs of the undergraduate students of dentistry.

Dr. R Rathy

Vice Principal, Professor & Head

Department of Oral Pathology & Microbiology

Azeezia College of Dental Sciences &Research,

Meeyannoor, Kollam, Kerala, India

Contents

Primary Teeth 1
Introduction to Dental Anatomy 5
Permanent Maxillary Teeth 23
Permanent Mandibular Teeth 47
Differences Between Teeth 69
Mastication & Deglutition 79
Occlusion 87
Oral Histology 93
Bibiography 232

Primary Teeth

MAIN QUESTION

Q1) Describe the macroscopic and microscopic differences between primary and permanent teeth.

Answer –

Macroscopic differences

Sl. No.	Primary teeth	Permanent teeth
1	Number – total 20 teeth.	Number – total 32 teeth.
2	Size – Overall smaller size	Size – Overall larger size
3	Enamel is thinner, more opaque and whiter, thus imparting a white hue to the crown.	Enamel is thicker, less opaque and less white, imparting yellowish white colour to the crown.
4	Mamelons are absent.	Mamelons are seen in newly erupted incisors.
5	Crowns markedly constricted in the cervical region.	Crowns less constricted in the cervical region.
6	Both anterior and posterior teeth have noticeable buccal cervical ridges.	The anterior and posterior teeth have less noticeable buccal cervical ridges.
7	Anterior teeth have greater mesiodistal width than the cervicoincisal crown height.	Mesiodistal width in anterior teeth is lesser than the cervicoincisal crown height
8	In relation to the height of their crowns, front teeth have greater roots. They are also flatter mesiodistally	In connection to the height of their crowns, front teeth have smaller roots. They are round.
9	Compared to first molars, second molars are substantially larger.	Compared to first molars, second molars are smaller.
10	Occlusal table in posterior teeth are narrower bucco-lingually.	Occlusal table in posterior teeth are wider bucco-lingually.
11	Premolars and third molars are absent	Premolars and third molars are present.
12	There is a short root trunk. The cervical line is closer towards the furcation.	Root trunk is broader. The cervical line is far from the furcation.
13	Molar roots are longer, thinner, more flare out beyond the crown outline to accommodate the developing premolar.	Molar roots are more substantial, longer and do not flare out.
14	Compared to first molars, second molar roots are more flared.	First molar roots more flared compared to second molars.

| 15 | Teeth exhibit very little variation in morphology | Teeth show more variation in morphology. |

Microscopic differences

Sl. No.	Primary teeth	Permanent teeth
1	They are less mineralized and wear off faster.	They are more mineralized and resistant to wearing.
2	Perikymata are absent.	Perikymata are present.
3	Pulp chambers are larger with high pulp horns.	Pulp chambers are smaller with not too high pulp horns.
4	Pulp canals are thinner.	Pulp canals are wider.
5	The cervical region's enamel rods slant in occlusal or incisal direction.	In the cervical area, enamel rods slope in a cervical orientation.
6	Enamel is relatively thin.	Enamel is relatively thick.
7	Interglobular dentin is absent.	It is present.
8	Less regular dentinal tubules.	More consistent.
9	Wide apical foramen.	Narrow foramen.
10	Every tooth has a neonatal line.	Limited to first molars.

****

SHORT NOTES

Q1) Importance of deciduous / primary teeth.

Answer –

- Deciduous teeth are essential for the proper development and growth of the jaws.
- It acts as natural space maintainers for the eruption of permanent successors. If they are lost prematurely, it leads to the migration of the adjacent deciduous teeth in the space thus created. This results in insufficient space for the erupting successors, leading to malocclusion. Sometimes they may not erupt.
- Normal occlusal relation in the permanent teeth depends on adequate spacing in the deciduous dentition.
- They help to maintain normal facial appearance.
- Mastication of food.
- Anterior teeth are essential for pronunciation of certain words.

****

Introduction to Dental Anatomy

SHORT NOTES

Q1) Tooth numbering systems.

Answer – An important part in dental practice is to record, preserve and retrieve dental data. Tooth notation or numbering systems are a means for communication. Therefore it is important to follow a coding system or numbering system for the teeth.

Three different tooth numbering schemes exist.

a) Universal numbering system.
b) Zsigmondy-Palmer system of notation.
c) Federation Dentaire Internationale (FDI) system.

UNIVERSAL NUMBERING SYSTEM

- This method of tooth numbering was accepted by the American Dental Association.
- Permanent teeth are numbered from 1-32 that begin with right maxillary third molar.

Upper Right quadrant								Upper Left quadrant							
1	2	3	4	5	6	7	8	9	10	11	12	13	14	15	16
32	31	30	29	28	27	26	25	24	23	22	21	20	19	18	17
Lower Right quadrant								Lower Left quadrant							

Examples: Permanent central incisor of the maxillary right side – 8

Permanent maxillary left second molar – 15

- Deciduous teeth are denoted in alphabets from A to T (all capital letters), starting with the maxillary second molar in the right quadrant.

Upper Right quadrant					Upper Left quadrant				
A	B	C	D	E	F	G	H	I	J
T	S	R	Q	P	O	N	M	L	K
Lower Right quadrant					Lower Left quadrant				

Examples: Deciduous central incisor in the right maxilla – E

Deciduous maxillary left second molar – J

Advantages of universal system –

a) System is simple to understand.
b) Each tooth has its own number or alphabet.
c) The left and right teeth, the upper and lower teeth, are assigned different numerals or alphabets.
d) Compatible for use with the computer key board and easy to type.
e) It can be communicated verbally.

Disadvantages of universal system –

a) Difficult to remember the number or alphabet of each tooth.
b) Difficulty in visually identifying each tooth.
c) More chances of error.
d) Time consuming.

ZSIGMONDY-PALMER SYSTEM

- This system divides each arch into two quadrants. A symbol represents each quadrant. The horizontal line indicates the occlusal plane that divides the upper and lower arches, while the vertical line indicates the patient's midline. Both permanent and deciduous teeth have the same symbol.

    Maxillary right and left quadrants   –   R⏊ ⏊L

    Mandibular right and left quadrants –   R⏉ ⏉L

- Permanent dentition – The teeth in each quadrant are numbered 1 to 8 that begin with the central incisor anteriorly and end at third molar posteriorly.

Upper Right quadrant							Upper Left quadrant						
8	7	6	5	4	3	2	1	1	2	3	4	5	6	7	8
8	7	6	5	4	3	2	1	1	2	3	4	5	6	7	8
Lower Right quadrant							Lower Left quadrant						

Examples: Maxillary right central incisor – 1⏌

Maxillary left second molar – ⏌7

Deciduous dentition -- The teeth in each quadrant is alphabetically labeled from A to E (all capital letters) that begins with the central incisor anteriorly and end at second molar posteriorly.

Upper Right quadrant					Upper Left quadrant				
E	D	C	B	A	A	B	C	D	E
E	D	C	B	A	A	B	C	D	E
Lower Right quadrant					Lower Left quadrant				

Examples: Maxillary right central incisor – A ⏌

　　　　　Mandibular right canine – C ⏋

Advantages of Z-P system

a) It is simple to follow.
b) Symbols are same for both dentitions.
c) It gives a graphical image of dentition.

Disadvantages of Z-P system

a) Difficult to use in computers as typing the symbols is difficult and time consuming.
b) Verbal communication is not possible.
c) The same number/letter used for a tooth may create confusion whether it is a left/right side or upper/lower teeth.

FDI NOTATION SYSTEM / TWO-DIGIT SYSTEM

- The most recent notation system is FDI system adopted by the International Dental Federation.
- It is also called a two-digit system because it numbers both the quadrant as well as the teeth. The first digit denotes the quadrant and second digit denotes the tooth.

  Quadrants in permanent dentition are numbered from 1 to 4 which are...

  ✓ Right maxillary   (1)
  ✓ Left maxillary   (2)
  ✓ Left mandibular   (3)
  ✓ Right mandibular   (4)

- According to the Zsigmondy Palmer system, the teeth in each quadrant are indicated by numbers 1 to 8, starting from the central incisor in the midline and moving posteriorly to the third molar. But here there is an additional number representing the quadrant.

- E.g. 1-centralincisor; 2- lateral incisor; 3- canine; 4- first premolar and so on.

Upper Right quadrant	Upper Left quadrant
18 17 16 15 14 13 12 11	21 22 23 24 25 26 27 28
48 47 46 45 44 43 42 41	31 32 33 34 35 36 37 38
Lower Right quadrant	Lower Left quadrant

Examples

12 – Permanent right maxillary lateral incisor.

34 – Permanent mandibular left first premolar.

In deciduous dentition, quadrants are similarly numbered from 5 to 8

- ✓ Right maxillary   (5)
- ✓ Left maxillary   (6)
- ✓ Left mandibular   (7)
- ✓ Right mandibular   (8)
- According to the Zsigmondy Palmer system, the teeth in each quadrant are indicated by numbers 1 to 5, beginning with the central incisor in the midline and moving posteriorly to the second molar. But here there is an additional number representing the quadrant.

Upper Right quadrant	Upper Left quadrant
55 54 53 52 51	61 62 63 64 65
85 84 83 82 81	71 72 73 74 75
Lower Right quadrant	Lower Left quadrant

Examples

65 – Deciduous maxillary left second molar.

83 – Deciduous mandibular right canine.

- In two-digit system, each tooth is pronounced as separate numbers and not as a whole. The permanent maxillary right lateral incisor for instance, is pronounced one-two rather than twelve.

Advantages

  a) Widely used system in the majority of the world.
  b) Simple to understand and teach.
  c) Easy to communicate.
  d) Can be used in computers and easy to type.
  e) Prevents errors when differentiating right and left sides and upper and lower arches.

****

Q2) Universal notation system for teeth.

Answer – An important part in dental practice is to record, preserve and retrieve dental data. Tooth notation or numbering systems are a means for communication. Therefore it is important to follow a coding system or numbering system for the teeth.

- Refer section 'Universal notation system' in short notes Q1 of chapter 'Introduction to dental anatomy'.

****

Q3) FDI notation system.

Answer – An important part in dental practice is to record, preserve and retrieve dental data. Tooth notation or numbering systems are a means for communication. Therefore it is important to follow a coding system or numbering system for the teeth.

- Refer section 'FDI notation system' in short notes Q1 of chapter 'Introduction to dental anatomy'.

****

Q4) Dental formula.

Answer – Human beings are diphyodonts and have two sets of dentition in their life span – deciduous and permanent teeth.

Each quadrant's tooth number and class are indicated by a dental formula. The initial letter of each tooth's name serves as a representation. For instance, Premolars are denoted by P, molars by M, canines by C, and incisors by I. Each letter has a line running horizontally after it. The upper arch's tooth count is above the line, while the lower arch's tooth count is below it. The formula applies only to one side of the arch.

- The twenty deciduous teeth are separated into three classes: molars, canines, and incisors. Each quadrant contains two incisors, one canine along with two molars.

Dental formula for deciduous teeth on one side of midline.

$$I \frac{2}{2} - C \frac{1}{1} - M \frac{2}{2} -$$

- There are thirty-two permanent teeth, divided into four groups: canines, incisors, molars, and premolars. Each quadrant contains three molars, two premolars, one canine and two incisors.
Dental formula for permanent teeth on one side of midline.

$$I \frac{2}{2} - C \frac{1}{1} - PM \frac{2}{2} - M \frac{3}{3} -$$

****

Q5) Set trait, arch traits, class traits, type traits.

Answer --Traits are characteristics or features that are used to differentiate or identify teeth. These are....
1. Set trait
2. Arch trait
3. Class trait
4. Type trait

SET TRAITS

Set traits are features that differentiate teeth of deciduous dentition from that of permanent dentition. *For e.g.* i) The size of primary teeth is smaller than that of permanent teeth; ii) Compared to permanent teeth, primary teeth are more white.

ARCH TRAITS

Arch traits are the features that help to differentiate between the maxillary and mandibular teeth. *For e.g.* i) Mandibular posteriors (molars) have two roots, where as maxillary have three ii) Maxillary posteriors are wider buccolingually whereas mandibular posteriors are wider mesiodistally.

CLASS TRAITS

Class traits are the features that are used to group the teeth into four classes, namely incisors, canines, premolars and molars. *For e.g.* (i) Canines have a pointed cusp, while incisors have a straight incisal edge. (ii) Molars have three to five flattened cusps, while premolars have two or three.

TYPE TRAITS

The characteristics that distinguish teeth of the same class -- central and lateral incisors, first and second premolars, first, second, and third molars, etc -- are known as type attributes. *For e.g.* i) the incisal edge of the maxillary lateral incisor is curved with more rounded mesial and distal incisal angles while that of the maxillary central incisor is straight. ii) In contrast to second premolar, maxillary first premolar has two roots. iii) While the buccal and palatal cusps of the second premolar are the same height, the palatal cusp of the maxillary first premolar is 1 mm shorter.

****

Q6) Stages of dentition.

Answer – *There are three stages in human dentition……*

- Primary dentition phase (6 months - 6 years)
- Mixed dentition phase (6 - 12 years)
- Permanent dentition phase (12 years - above)

Deciduous dentition period

- Deciduous dentition period start from the time of eruption of first primary tooth, usually the mandibular central incisor at around six months of age and lasts until the emergence of the first permanent tooth around six years of age.
- During this time, the oral cavity has only deciduous teeth.

Mixed dentition period

- The term "mixed dentition period" refers to the presence of both primary and permanent teeth throughout this time.
- As the original teeth gradually fall out, the permanent erupts.
- The mixed dentition stage commences with the emergence of mandibular first molar and central incisor in the oral cavity by about the age of 6. The stage ends by around the age of 12 when the last primary tooth is shed.

Permanent dentition period

- When all of the permanent teeth erupt, the permanent dentition phase begins.
- There are no deciduous teeth during this period.

****

Q7) Line angles and point angles.

Answer – These are only descriptive terms used to describe the crown; there aren't any actual lines or angles there identify a position on a tooth.

Line angle

- On a tooth, the line angle is the angle created where two surfaces join.
- The names of the two surfaces that unite are combined to give it its name. For instance, the mesiobuccal line angle is the point where a tooth's buccal and mesial walls join.
- There are eight line angles in a posterior tooth compared to six in an anterior tooth.

Line angles on anterior teeth	*Line angles on posterior teeth*
Distolabial	Linguo-occlusal
Distolingual	Bucco-occlusal
Linguoincisal	Disto-occlusal
Mesiolabial	Mesiolingual
Labioincisal	Mesio-occlusal
Mesiolingual	Distolingual
	Distobuccal
	Mesiobuccal

Point angle

- The angle that is formed where three surfaces of a tooth meet on the crown is called point angle.
- It is named by combining the names of the three surfaces that join. e.g. the junction of mesial, labial and incisal walls of an anterior tooth is called mesiolabioincisalpoint angle.
- An anterior tooth has four point angles, while a posterior tooth has four.

Point angles on anterior teeth	*Point angles on posterior teeth*
Mesiolabioincisal	Mesiobucco-occlusal
Distolabioincisal	Distobucco-occlusal
Mesiolinguoincisal	Mesiolinguo-occlusal
Distolinguoincisal	Distolinguo-occlusal

Q8) Cusp, ridge, fossa, cingulum.

Answer –

CUSP

- Cusps are pointed, raised projections on the occlusal table of posterior teeth.
- It is conical or pyramidal.

- Number of cusps varies for each tooth. e.g., Except for the mandibular second premolar which has three cusps, other premolars have two cusps. All molars typically have four cusps, while maxillary and mandibular first molars have five.

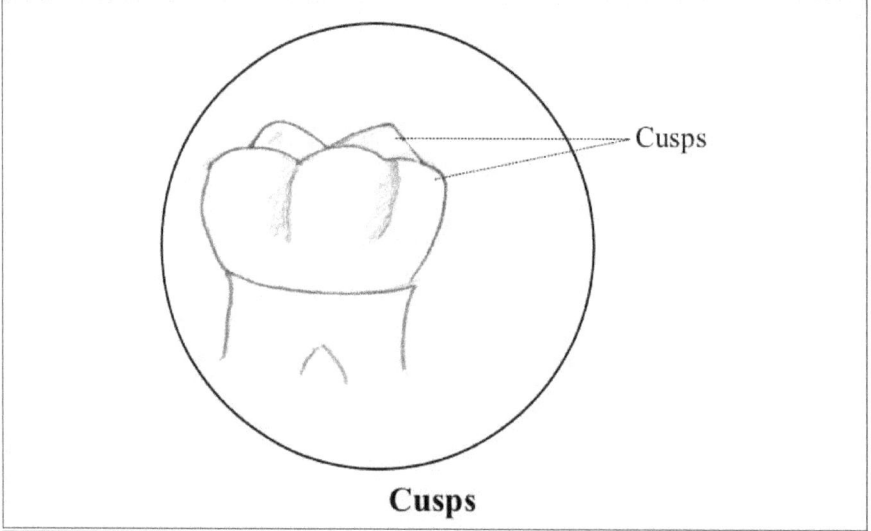

Cusps

RIDGE

- Ridge is an even elevation on the tooth surface.
- Its location determines its name.

Buccal ridge

- On the buccal surface of premolars and molars (posterior teeth), there is an even elevation known as the buccal ridge. It extends to the cervical line from the cusp tip.

Labial ridge

- Labial ridge is an even elevation that runs on the labial surface of canines (anterior teeth). It runs from the cusp tip till the cervical line.

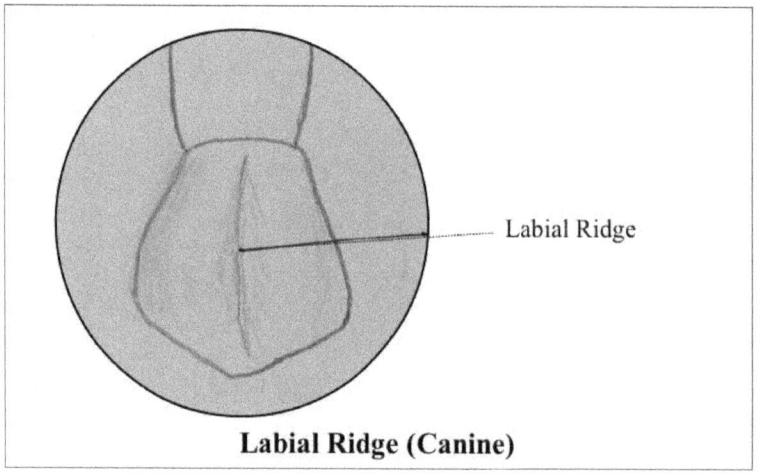

Labial Ridge (Canine)

Lingual ridge

- The lingual surface of the premolar as well molar has a ridge on it. It reaches the cervical line from the tip of the lingual cusp. In case of canines, the lingual cusp ridge runs on the lingual surface, dividing the lingual fossa into two small fossae.

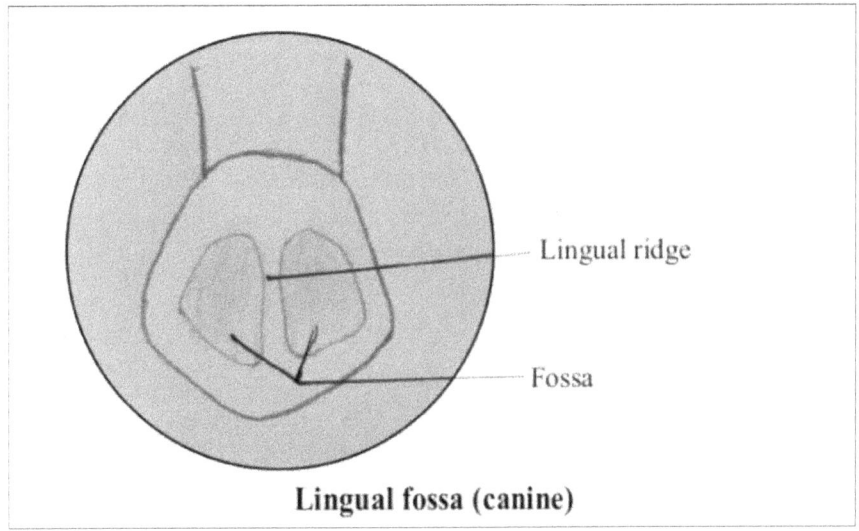

Lingual fossa (canine)

Cervical ridge

- In the cervical third of the buccal surface of the crown, there is a ridge that runs mesiodistally. It is a feature of every primary tooth. On deciduous maxillary and mandibular first molars, it is more prominent.

Incisal ridge

- Every incisor has an incisal ridge on its incisal face. It runs in mesiodistal direction.

Marginal ridge

- Marginal ridge is a rounded elevation of enamel that form the mesial and distal boundaries of lingual surfaces of all anterior teeth and mesial and distal boundaries of occlusal surface of all posterior teeth.

Triangular ridge

- The triangle ridge is a linear elevation that runs from the premolar and molar cusp tips to the center of the occlusal surface. Each cusp has a single triangular ridge. They are named according to the cusp they belong, e.g., triangular ridge of buccal cusp of maxillary second premolar.

Transverse ridge

- It is a ridge formed when the opposing cusp's triangular ridges joins.

Oblique ridge

- It is a ridge that obliquely traverses the occlusal surface. It is formed by joining the triangular ridges of the maxillary first molar's mesiopalatal cusp and distobuccal cusp.
- Only maxillary molars have an oblique ridge. On permanent maxillary first molars, it is most prominent. The permanent maxillary second and third molars may have it. The deciduous maxillary second molar also has it.

FOSSA

- An uneven cavity or depression on the lingual surface of the anterior teeth and the occlusal surface of the posterior teeth is called a fossa. Its location determines its name.

    Types
    - ✓ Lingual fossa
    - ✓ Central fossa
    - ✓ Triangular fossa
    - ✓ Canine fossa

Lingual fossa

All of the anterior teeth have it on their lingual surfaces. It is delimited by marginal ridges on both the mesial along with distal sides respectively. Furthermore, it is encircled by the cusp slopes on canines and the incisal ridge on incisors. It is shallow in lower anteriors than in the upper anteriors.

Central fossa

The maxillary and mandibular molar's central fossa, resides in the middle of their occlusal surfaces. There is a central pit in it and various grooves converge at its depth.

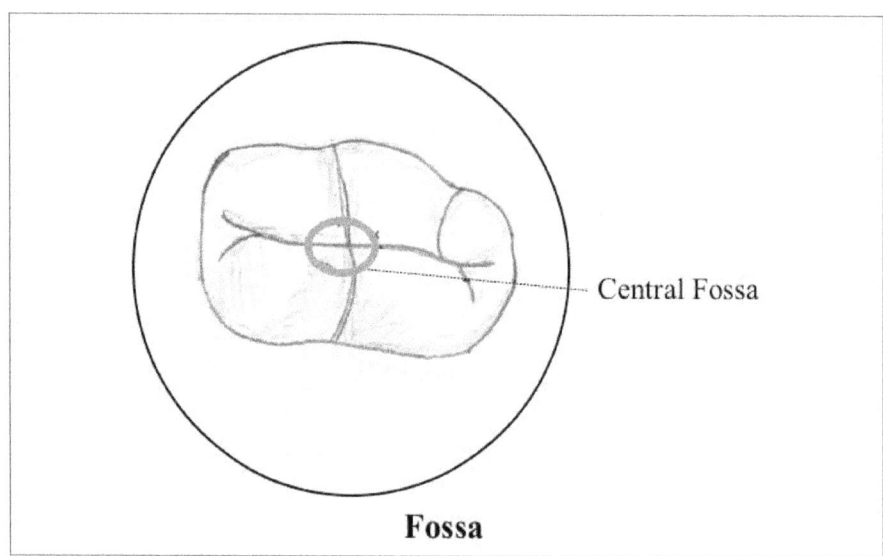

Fossa

Triangular fossa

Premolar and molar occlusal surfaces have a triangular fossa. Both the distal and mesial triangular fossae are situated mesially to the distal marginal ridge and distally to the mesial marginal ridge respectively. The reason for its name is that it resembles a triangle. The pit is the triangle's apex, while the peripheral ridge is its base.

Canine fossa

It is also called as mesial development depression. It is the characteristic feature of maxillary first premolar only and is located on its mesial surface. It is believed to be produced due to the pressure applied by the distal aspect of maxillary canine as it develops earlier than the first premolar and hence the name canine fossa.

CINGULUM

- The convexity or bulge on the maxillary and mandibular lingual surfaces in the cervical third of anteriors that is oriented mesiodistally is known as the cingulum.

- It is most prominent on the maxillary permanent canine.

- It represents the lingual lobe of the tooth.

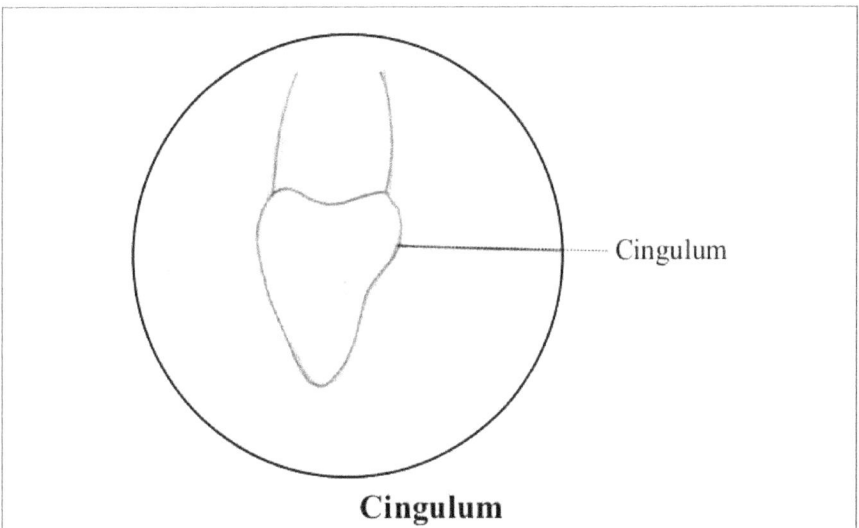

Cingulum

Q9) Grooves.

Answer–Grooves can be defined as a sharp, long or short lines or depression on a tooth. They indicate the union of primary parts i.e. lobes.

Grooves are named according to their location, e.g.

a) The buccal surface of the maxillary and mandibular molars crowns possesses a *buccal developmental groove* that set apart the buccal cusps.

b) The lingual surface of the maxillary and mandibular molars crowns contains the *lingual developmental groove*. The lingual cusps are separated by it.

c) In premolar and molars, *central developmental groove* is located in the middle of their occlusal surfaces. It divides the lingual and buccal cusps. It runs mesiodistally from the mesial to the distal pit.

Supplemental grooves

- These are tiny, uneven grooves on the tooth's occlusal surface that are less prominent.

Developmental groove on the mesial marginal ridge of maxillary first premolar

- A well formed developmental groove is found crossing the mesial marginal ridge of maxillary first premolar only. This groove is continuous with the central developmental groove on the occlusal surface. After crossing the marginal ridge, it runs a short distance on the mesial surface and terminates at a short distance cervical to the mesial marginal ridge.

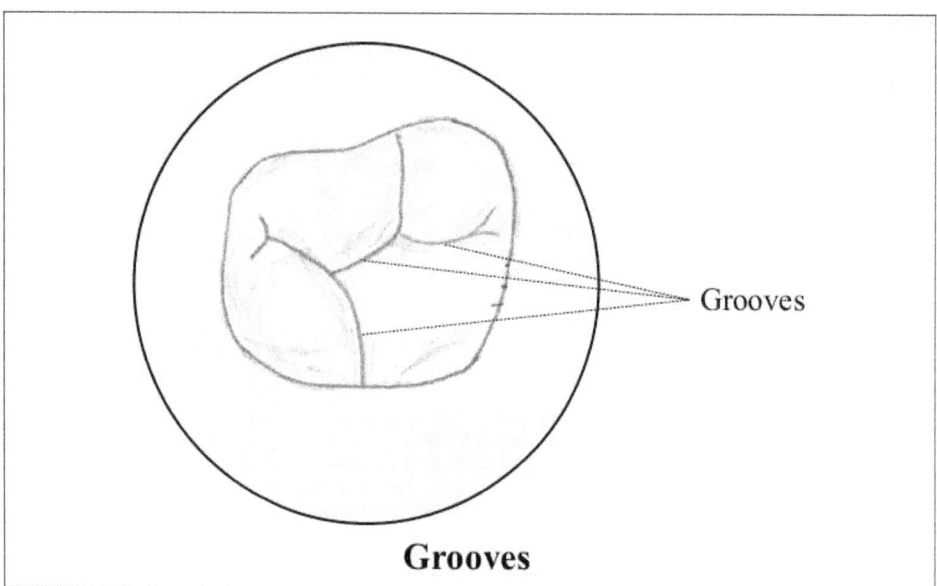

Q10) Contact areas

Q) Contact point and embrasures.

Answer –

Contact area / Contact point

- The contact point, also known as the contact area, is the location on the proximal surface (mesial or distal) where two neighboring teeth contact.
- Contact point is present in anterior teeth and contact area in posterior teeth.

- If there is no contact between the adjacent teeth, then the space between them is called *diastema*.
- Except for the maxillary and mandibular third molars, which have only one contact area on the mesial side, every tooth has two contact points or areas: one on the mesial side and one on the distal side.
- Proper contact between adjacent teeth is important as it prevents food accumulation in between the teeth. Food deposition may result in gingivitis and ultimately lead to periodontitis.
- Position of the contact point / area can be viewed from the labial/buccal sides or from incisal/occlusal sides.

Embrasure

- Embrasure is also called as interproximal space.
- Interproximal embrasures underneath the contact point are filled by interdental papilla.
- The space above the contact point/area towards the incisal or occlusal side is respectively called incisal/occlusal embrasures.
- During mastication, the embrasure facilitates food passage and keeps it from being driven into the contact region.

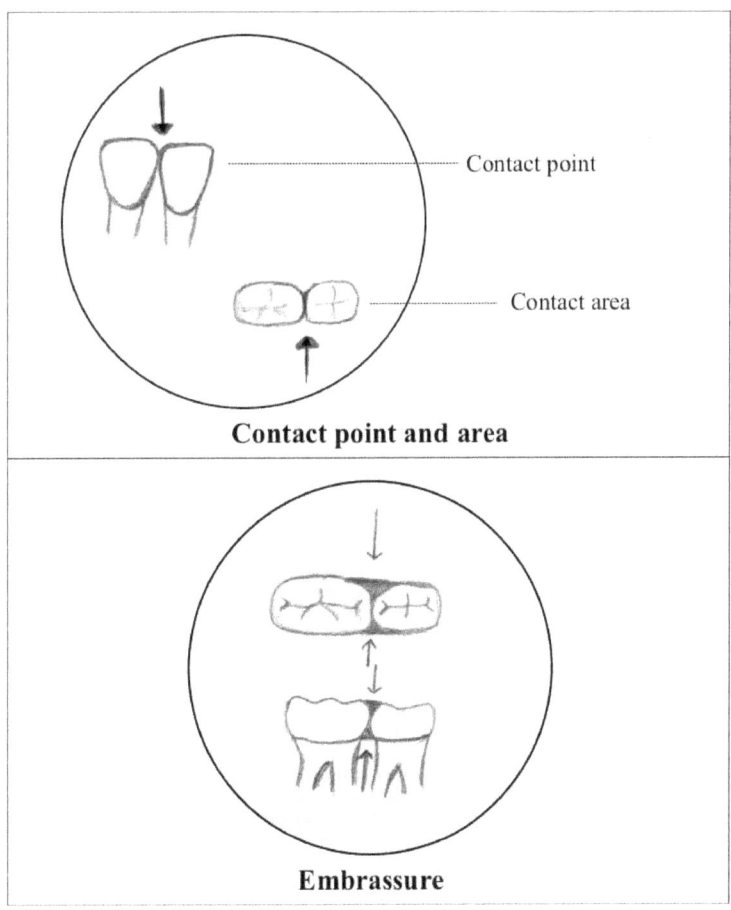

Contact point and area

Embrassure

Q11) Lobe

Answer --Lobe is a primary part from which the crown portion of a tooth develops. Once crown formation is complete, the lobe persists as cusps and mamelons.

- At least four lobes are involved in the development of a permanent tooth.
- Four lobes -- mesial, labial, distal and lingual are involved in development of anterior teeth. Lingual lobe forms the cingulum.
- Except mandibular second premolar, all premolars develop from mesial, buccal, distal, and lingual lobes.
- Mesial, buccal, distal, mesiolingual, and distolingual lobes develop into mandibular second premolar.
- Maxillary and mandibular first molars develop from five lobes. The other molars develop from four lobes.

Q12) Mamelons

Answer –Mamelons are three spherical elevations located on the incisal ridge of newly erupted incisors. They indicate the three labial lobes of the crown region during development. They require no treatment. Once the tooth gets functionality, the mamelons are eroded away, resulting in a straight incisal ridge. They are present only in the permanent incisors and not present in primary teeth.

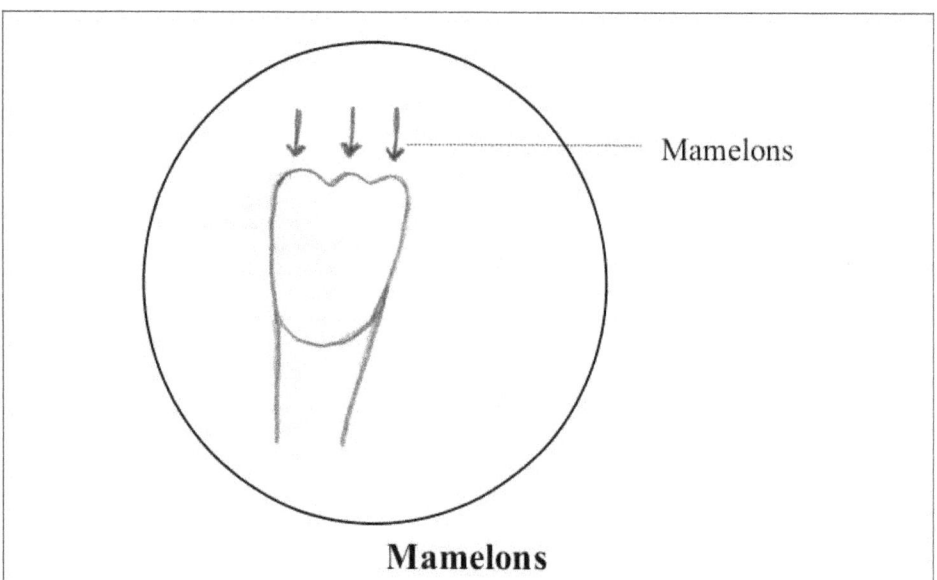

Mamelons

Q13) Line angles and point angles on posterior teeth.

Answer –

They are just descriptive terms that denote a specific location on a tooth; the crown itself does not have any lines or angles.

Line angle

- The angle made at the junction of two surfaces on a tooth is referred to as a line angle.
- It is marked by combining the names of the two junctional surfaces. The junction of the mesial and buccal walls of a tooth is referred to as the mesiobuccal line angle.
- There exist eight line angles on the posterior tooth.

Line angles on posterior teeth
Distolingual
Distobuccal
Mesiobuccal
Disto-occlusal
Bucco-occlusal
Mesiolingual
Linguo-occlusal
Mesio-occlusal

Point angle

- The angle that is formed where three surfaces of a tooth meet on the crown is called point angle.
- The names of the three surfaces that join are combined to give it its name. For instance, the mesiobuccoocclusal point angle is the junction of a posterior tooth's mesial, buccal, and occlusal surfaces.
- There are four point angles on the posterior tooth.

Point angles on posterior teeth
Distolinguo-occlusal
Mesiolinguo-occlusal
Distobucco-occlusal
Mesiobucco-occlusal

Q14) Line angles and point angles of anterior teeth.

Answer –

- These are only descriptive terms that denote a location on a tooth; crown itself does not have any actual lines or angles.

Line angle

- On a tooth, the line angle is the angle formed where two surfaces join.
- It is named by combining the names of the two surfaces that join. e.g., the junction of mesial and labial surfaces of an anterior tooth is called mesiolabial line angle.
- There exist six line angles on an anterior tooth.

Line angles on anterior teeth
Labioincisal
Mesiolingual
Distolingual
Mesiolabial
Distolabial
Linguoincisal

Point angle

- Point angle is the angle formed on a tooth's crown where three of its surfaces meet.
- It is named by combining the names of the three surfaces that join. e.g., the junction of mesial, labial and incisal surfaces of an anterior tooth is called mesiolabioincisal point angle.
- Anterior tooth possess four point angles, while posterior tooth also has four point angles.

Point angles on anterior teeth
Mesiolinguoincisal
Distolabioincisal
Distolinguoincisal
Mesiolabioincisal

Permanent Maxillary Teeth

CENTRAL INCISOR

Q1) Describe the morphological aspects of permanent maxillary central incisor.

Answer –

INTRODUCTION

- The maxillary central incisors are two in number, located on either side of the imaginary midline.
- The maxillary and mandibular central incisors are the only teeth in the dental arches that have their mesial surfaces in contact.
- It has a greatest mesiodistal width than any other anterior teeth.

TOOTH NOTATION

- Universal system – 8 and 9
- Zsigmondy / Palmer system –   1 | 1
- FDI system – 11 and 21

FUNCTIONS

Maxillary incisors along with the mandibular incisors perform the following functions

1] They assist in cutting food material during mastication.

2] Helps in pronouncing certain words.

3] Supports the lip.

DETAILED DESCRIPTION FROM ALL ASPECTS

LABIAL ASPECT

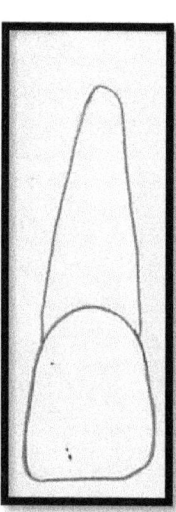

- Labial surface is smooth and convex.
- Mamelons may be observed on the incisal ridge of newly erupted teeth, but they are lost as the teeth become functional.
- *Crown outline* -- The tooth shows a trapezoidal shape, characterized by the smallest uneven side located at the neck (cervix) and the longest uneven side at the incisal edge. The mesial outline exhibits reduced convexity, with the crest of curvature located in the incisal third or near to the mesioincisal angle. The distal outline is more convex, with the crest of curvature located at the junction of the incisal and middle thirds.
- Mesioincisal angle is sharp compared to the distoincisal angle.
- Typically incisal outline is straight.
- *Cervical line* – It is semicircular with the convexity towards the root apex.

- *Root* -- Root is cone-shaped with blunt apex. A line extending from the center of the root and crown normally aligns parallel to the mesial outline of the crown and root.

PALATAL ASPECT

- Compared to the smooth labial surface, the palatal surface has certain irregularities characterized by both convexities and concavities.
- Most of the palatal surface is occupied by a concave depression called '*lingual fossa*'. On either side of this fossa are the "mesial and distal marginal ridges."
- *Cervical line* -- It is same as seen from the labial aspect, exhibiting a semicircular shape with the convexity directed towards the root apex.
- *Cingulum* -- Below the cervical line lies a smooth convexity known as the '*cingulum*,' which extends mesiodistally, covering the entire cervical third of the crown.
- Both the root and the crown have lingual tapering.
- *Root* – It has a blunt apex and is shaped like a cone.

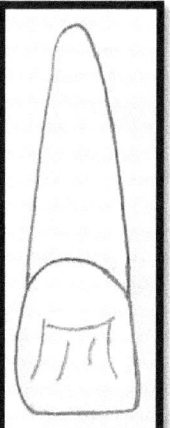

MESIAL ASPECT

- From the mesial aspect, the crown exhibits a triangular or wedge configuration, with the base positioned at the cervix and the apex at the incisal ridge.
- A line drawn across the center of the crown and the root will intersect the root apex and the incisal edge. It signifies that both the root apex and the incisal edge are aligned in a straight line.
- *Labial outline* – The crest of curvature is located in the cervical third labially. The labial outline is a little convex from the crest of curvature to the incisal edge.
- *Lingual outline* – The outline from the cervical line till the cingulum is convex. Below the cingulum, it becomes concave shape and subsequently becomes almost convex toward the incisal ridge.
- *Cervical line* – It curves sharply towards the incisal ridge. The curvature is greater on the mesial side than on the distal side.
- *Root* – The root has a blunt apex and a cone-like form.

DISTAL ASPECT

- The mesial and distal sides exhibit minimal differences.

- In comparison to the mesial aspect, the cervical line on this side exhibits a reduced curvature.

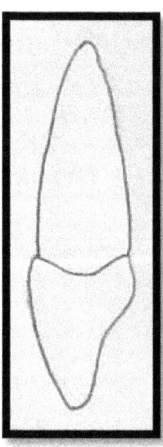

INCISAL ASPECT

- The crown exhibits a roughly triangular shape from the incisal aspect, with the labial surface constituting the base and the cingulum forming the apex.

- The crown has a wider mesiodistal width than labiolingual width.

- Incisal ridge is somewhat curved with the distoincisal angle being placed slightly lingual to the mesioincisal angle.

- The large cingulum, mesial and distal marginal ridges, and the concavity of the lingual fossa are observable from this aspect.

- From the incisal perspective, the crown overlays the root, making the root invisible from this aspect.

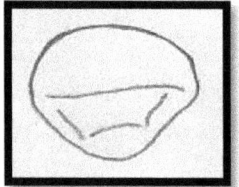

****

LATERAL INCISOR

MAIN QUESTION

Q1) Describe the morphology of permanent maxillary lateral incisor.

Answer –

INTRODUCTION

- The maxillary lateral incisor closely resembles the central incisor.
- Apart from the third molar, they exhibit more morphological variety than any other tooth in the mouth.

TOOTH NOTATION

- Universal system – 7 and 10
- Zsigmondy / Palmer system   2 | 2
- FDI system – 12 and 22

FUNCTIONS

Maxillary incisors along with the mandibular incisors carry out the following functions.

1] They are shearing or cutting teeth. They assist in cutting food material during mastication.

2] Helps in pronouncing certain words.

3] Supports the lip.

DETAILED DESCRIPTION FROM ALL ASPECTS

LABIAL ASPECT

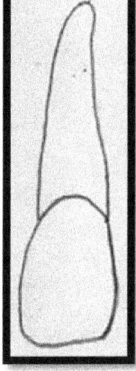

- Compared to the central incisor, the labial surface is smoother and more convex.
- *Crown outline* --The crown's outline is trapezoidal, the smallest uneven side at the neck (or cervix) of the tooth and the longest uneven side at the incisal edge. The crest of curvature on the mesial aspect is located at the junction of the middle third and incisal third, whereas distally it is in the center of the middle third. The mesial outline and mesioincisal angle are more rounded than those of the central incisor. The distal outline and distoincisal angle are significantly more rounded. The incisal edge contour is typically not linear, but is significantly inclined towards the distal side because of the greater rounding of the distoincisal angle.
- *Root* -- It has a sharp apex and cone-shaped.
- *Cervical line* – It is convex and semicircular.

PALATAL ASPECT

- The palatal surface exhibits irregularities characterized by both convexities and concavities.
- The "lingual fossa," a concavity that occupies majority of the palate surface, is bounded on both sides by "mesial and distal marginal ridges." The lingual fossa is more concave and distinctly defined than that of the central incisor. At times, prominent grooves can appear within the lingual fossa.
- *Cervical line* -- It is same as seen from the labial aspect i.e. convex in the direction of the root apex and semicircular.
- *Cingulum* -- Below the cervical line is a smooth convexity known as the 'cingulum,' which runs mesiodistally throughout the entire cervical third of the crown.
- Both crown and root show lingual tapering.
- *Root* – It has a pointed apex and is resembles a cone.

MESIAL ASPECT

- From the mesial aspect, the crown exhibits a triangular or wedge shape, with the base positioned at the cervical line and the tip at the incisal ridge.
- A line drawn through the center of the crown and the root will pass the root apex and the incisal edge. It indicates that both the root apex and the incisal edge are aligned in a straight line.
- *Labial outline* – It has a small convexity from the crest of curvature to the incisal ridge. The crest of curvature is located in the cervical third.
- *Lingual outline* – From the cervical line to the cingulum is convex. Below the cingulum, it becomes a concave shape and subsequently becomes slightly convex toward the incisal ridge.
- *Cervical line* – It sharply curves incisally. The curvature is greater on the mesial side than on the distal side.
- *Root* – It has a blunt apex and a cone-like form.

DISTAL ASPECT

- The characteristics from the distal aspect are similar to those observed from the mesial aspect.
- *Cervical line* – In comparison to the mesial side, the cervical line exhibits a reduced curvature.

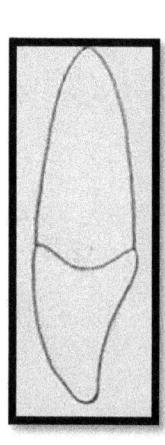

INCISAL ASPECT

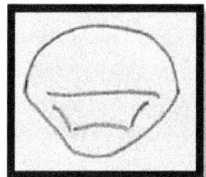

- The maxillary lateral incisor has a resemblance to the central incisor, with the exception of its size.
- The crown has a roughly triangular shape, with the base constituted by the labial surface and the apex defined by the cingulum.
- The teeth exhibit greater convexity both labially and lingually compared to the central incisor.
- The labiolingual dimension could be higher than the mesiodistal dimension.
- The incisal ridge has a small curvature, with the distoincisal angle positioned slightly lingual to the mesioincisal angle.
- This aspect shows the large cingulum, mesial and distal marginal ridges, and the concavity of the lingual fossa.
- From this perspective, the crown superimposes the root, making it invisible.

***

CANINE
MAIN QUESTION

Q1) Describe the morphological aspects of permanent maxillary canine.

Answer –

INTRODUCTION

- The maxillary arch has two canines, one in each quadrant. They are distal to the lateral incisor.
- Canines are described as *"corner stone"* of the dental arches.
- They are the longest teeth in the mouth with the exception of mandibular canine which may also be as long as that.
- Canines are held in the mouth for an extended duration for the following reasons.
  a) The surface area where periodontal ligament fibers can attach is increased due to long, wider root and a development groove.
  b) Smooth convex surface on crown helps for easy flushing of food debris.
  c) Their location in mouth facilitates proper cleaning.

FUNCTIONS

- ✓ Supports lips and facial musculature.
- ✓ Assists in cutting and tearing food.

- ✓ Guides occlusion.
- ✓ It acts as excellent abutments for fixed or removable prosthesis.

TOOTH NOTATION

- Universal system – 6 and 11
- Zsigmondy / Palmer system – 3⏐3
- FDI system – 13 and 23

DETAILED DESCRIPTION FROM ALL ASPECTS

LABIAL ASPECT

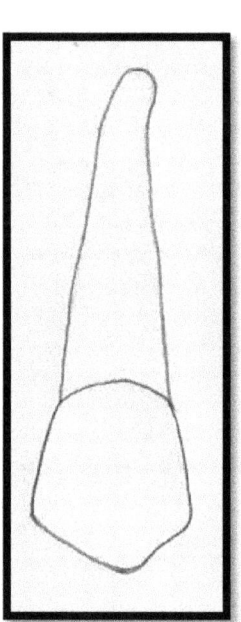

- The crown and root are thinner mesiodistally than those of the maxillary central incisor.
- *Cervical line* – It exhibits uniform convexity towards the root apex.
- *Labial surface* – The labial surface of the crown is smooth. The middle lobe is sufficiently developed to constitute the labial ridge. This ridge extends cervicoincisally at the center of the crown. A line drawn at the crest of this ridge, extending from the cervical line to the cusp tip, is inclined slightly mesially. The area mesial to this ridge displays convexity, while the distal area demonstrates concavity.
- *Mesial outline* -- It may exhibit convexity from the cervical line to the mesial contact area or may display minor concavity. The contact area mesially is located at the junction of the middle third and the incisal third.
- *Distal outline* – It is frequently concave between the cervical line and the distal contact region. The contact area distally is located near the center of the middle third of the crown.
- The canine possesses only one cusp. This cusp has two ridges: the shorter mesial ridge and the longer distal ridge. The angle formed by the cusp ridges is approximately 105 degrees.
- The cusp tip typically lies mesial to the line that bisects the crown mesiodistally.
- *Root* – It possesses a conical form, elongated and terminating in either a sharp or blunt apex. The apical part of the root has a distal curvature.

PALATAL ASPECT

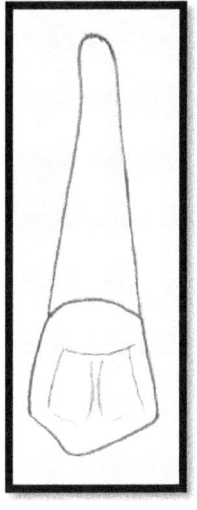

- Both crown and root show palatal tapering.
- *Cervical line* -- It has a more even convex curvature directed towards root apex.
- *Cingulum* – It is large and bulky. It may at times be pointed like a little cusp.
- *Fossa* -- Below to the cingulum is the lingual fossa, bordered by the mesial and distal marginal ridges.
- *Lingual ridge* -- At the center of the lingual fossa, a lingual ridge extends cervicoincisally from the cingulum to the cusp tip. The lingual ridge divides the lingual fossa into mesial and distal lingual fossae.
- *Root* – It possesses a conical shape, elongated and terminating in either a sharp or blunt apex.
- The palatal taper of the root shows developmental depression from this aspect.

MESIAL ASPECT

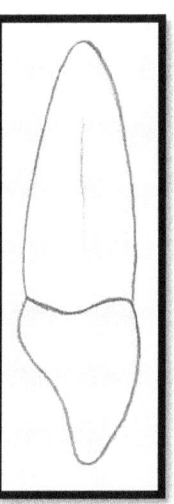

- From this aspect, the canine exhibits the functional shape of the anterior tooth.
- It shows more labiolingual measurement compared to all other anterior teeth.
- *Crown outline* – It possesses a triangular shape, with the base oriented towards the cervical line and the apex directed towards the cusp tip. The labial outline is smooth and convex from the cervical line to the cusp apex. The crest of curvature can be found in the cervical third on the labial side. The palatal outline in the cervical third is convex, becomes flat in the fossa, and return to convex in the incisal third. The crest of curvature is located in the center of cervical third.
- In this aspect, the cusp tip is observed to be positioned somewhat labial to the line that bisects the crown and root.
- *Cervical line* – It curves incisally.
- *Root* – It seems broad labiolingually. The labial and palatal outlines remain parallel till the middle third, after which they taper towards the apex. Developmental depression is observable on the root.

DISTAL ASPECT

- With a few exceptions, the distal and mesial aspects are nearly same.
- *Cervical line* – The curvature is not so much as compared to the mesial side.
- More concavity is visible on this surface, typically above the contact region.
- *Root* --The developmental depression is more prominent than on the mesial side.

INCISAL ASPECT

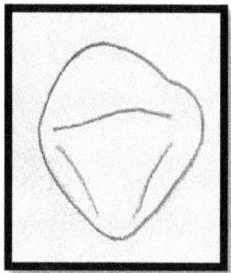

- From the incisal perspective, the crown exhibits mostly rhomboidal shape, with the corners of the rhombus formed by the elevations of the labial ridge, cingulum, and mesial and distal contact regions.
- Labiolingual dimension is greater than the mesiodistal dimension.
- The cusp tip seems to be positioned slightly labial to the line that bisects the crown labiolingually. The cusp tip is positioned mesial to the line that bisects the crown in a mesiodistal orientation.
- The mesial and distal cusp slopes often exhibit a straight course.
- The mesial half of the labial surface is convex, whereas the distal half is either flat or slightly concave.
- Prominent cingulum, lingual ridge, and mesial and distal marginal ridges are observable on palatal side.

****

FIRST PREMOLAR
MAIN QUESTION

Q1) Describe the morphological aspects of permanent maxillary first premolar.

Answer –

INTRODUCTION

- There are two maxillary first premolars: one on the left and one on the right.
- They are located before the second premolars and behind the canines.
- Premolars are named as such due to their position anterior to the molars.

FUNCTIONS

- Premolars assist canines in tearing and cutting the food into smaller pieces.
- Premolars together with the molars help in maintaining the vertical length of the face.

TOOTH NOTATION

- Universal system – 5 and 12

- Zsigmondy / Palmer system – 4ǀ4

- FDI system – 14 and 24

DETAILED DESCRIPTION FROM ALL ASPECTS

BUCCAL ASPECT

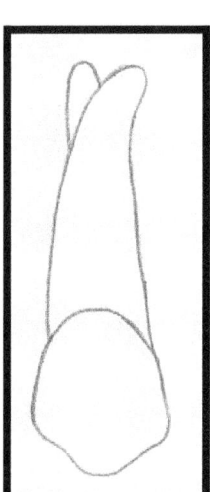

- The crown has a trapezoidal shape whose longest uneven side being occlusally and shortest uneven side cervically.
- The mesial outline from the cervical line to the mesial contact area is slightly concave. The contact area is broad. It is nearly at the center of the middle third.
- The distal outline is straight from the cervical margin to the distal contact region. The distal contact region is wider than on the mesial side. It is located near the junction of the middle and occlusal thirds.
- From this perspective, it resembles a canine due to its elongated buccal cusp with a pointed apex. The mesial slope of the cusp is linear and elongated, but the distal slope is shorter and more curved. The buccal cusp tip is positioned distal to the line that bisects the crown mesiodistally.
- The buccal surface of the crown is convex, with a well-developed middle buccal lobe that constitutes the *'buccal ridge.'* This ridge extends from the cusp tip to the cervical line. A shallow depression is observed on both sides of this ridge.
- The root is conical, elongated, and tapered, terminating in a blunt apex. The apical part of the root has a distal curvature.

PALATAL ASPECT

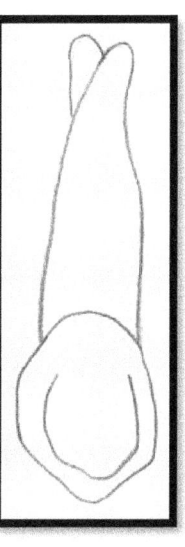

- The crown and the root taper palatally. Hence some of the mesial and the distal regions of the crown and root are visible from this aspect.
- The palatal cusp is narrower in the mesiodistal dimension than the buccal cusp. It is smooth and round. The cusp tip is sharp, with the mesial and distal slopes converging at right angle. The *'lingual ridge'* may also be observed on the palatal cusp, extending from the lingual cusp tip to the cervical line.
- The palatal cusp is shorter than the buccal cusp, allowing for visibility of the tips of both cusps together with their mesial and distal slopes.
- The mesial and distal outlines of the crown are convex and continue with the mesial and distal slopes of the palatal cusp.
- The root tapers uniformly from the cervical line and terminates in a blunt apex.

MESIAL ASPECT

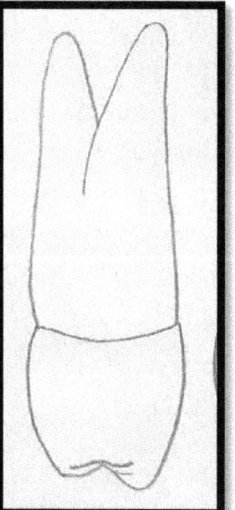

- From this aspect, the crown displays the trapezoidal shape that characterizes posterior teeth, with the largest uneven side located cervically and the shortest occlusally.
- All posterior maxillary teeth are characterized by cusp tips that lie well within the confines of the root trunk.
- The buccal and lingual outlines are smooth and convex from the cervical line to the cusp tip.
- The crest of curvature buccally is located at the junction of the cervical and middle thirds, whereas palatally it is situated at the midpoint of the middle third.
- Both cusps are visible from this perspective, with the buccal cusp being larger than the palatal cusp and longer in length by approximately one millimeter.
- The mesial marginal ridge is located at the intersection of the middle and occlusal thirds.
- The cervical line is less prominent than that of the anterior teeth.
- This perspective discloses both roots. Root bifurcation typically occurs at approximately fifty percent of the root length. Developmental depression is observed on the root extending from the canine fossa.

Two characteristic features found on the first premolar's mesial surface helps to distinguish it from the second premolar.

1. **Mesial developmental depression** – It is sometimes referred commonly as canine fossa. On the mesial surface, this depression it is situated just beneath the mesial contact area. The condition is thought to be the result from the pressure applied by the developing canine.
2. **Developmental groove on mesial marginal ridge** – The first premolar's mesial marginal ridge is crossed by a distinct groove *(mesial marginal developmental groove)*. This groove runs a short distance on the mesial surface, traverses over the mesial marginal ridge and continues with the central groove.

DISTAL ASPECT

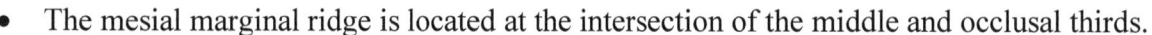

- Although the distal and mesial aspects are nearly identical, they differ in the following views.
  a) On the distal side, the cervical line has less curvature.
  b) No groove crosses the distal marginal ridge.
  c) Root trunk is flat.
  d) Compared to the mesial side, the bifurcation begins at a more apical position.
  e) On the distal surface, there is no canine fossa.

OCCLUSAL ASPECT

- The crown exhibits bucco-lingual tapering.
- The occlusal table resembles a hexagonal shape with six sides. The six surfaces are mesiobuccal, distobuccal, mesiopalatal, distopalatal, mesial, and distal.
- Each maxillary posterior tooth possesses a crown that is wider bucco-lingually than mesiodistally (characteristic feature of all maxillary posterior teeth).
- In comparison to the distal contact area, the mesial contact region appears to be positioned more buccally.
- The occlusal surface is surrounded by cusp ridges and marginal ridges.

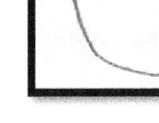

1. **Cusp ridges** – Distobuccal, distopalatal, mesiobuccal, and mesiopalatal are the four cusp ridges. The cusp ridges of the buccal cusp (distobuccal and mesiobuccal) are in a straight line. An acute angle is formed by the distobuccal cusp ridge and the distal marginal ridge, while a right angle is formed at the junction of mesiobuccal cusp ridge and mesial marginal ridge.
2. **Triangular ridges** – These two triangular ridges are called buccal and palatal triangular ridges, and named after the cusps on which they are found. The noticeable *buccal triangular ridge* extends from midway between the central groove and the buccal cusp tip. Less noticeable is the lingual triangular ridge that extends from the central groove to the tip for the palatal cusp.
3. **Transverse ridge** – Buccal and palatal triangular ridges join to form transverse ridge.
4. **Marginal ridges** – The mesial marginal ridge is shorter buccolingually than the distal marginal ridge. The mesial marginal ridge is crossed by the mesial developmental groove.

- *Grooves* – The occlusal surface is comparatively smooth, lacking any additional grooves. The *central developmental groove* symmetrically bisects the occlusal surface in a bucco-lingual direction. This groove extends at the base of the central fossa on the occlusal surface, originating from the distal pit, traversing to the mesial triangular fossa, and then crossing the mesial marginal ridge to persist as the *mesial marginal developmental groove*. This groove continues down the mesial marginal ridge and terminates on the mesial surface of the crown. Two additional grooves connect with the central groove immediately within the mesial and distal marginal ridges. These are referred to as the *mesiobuccal developmental groove* and the *distobuccal developmental groove*. At the junction of these grooves with the central groove, there exist deep depressions known as *mesial and distal developmental pits*.
- **Fossae** -- The *mesial triangular fossa* is a triangular depression located just distal to the mesial marginal ridge that houses the mesiobuccal groove. The triangular fossa, located directly mesial to the distal marginal ridge is the *distal triangular fossa* that houses the distobuccal groove.
- **Cusp** -- Compared to the buccal cusp, the lingual cusp is narrower, smaller and has a sharper point.

****

SECOND PREMOLAR
MAIN QUESTION

Q1) Describe the morphological aspects of permanent maxillary second premolar.

Answer –

INTRODUCTION

- First and second premolars resemble very closely.
- Unlike first premolar it has a single root.

TOOTH NOTATION

- Universal system – 4 and 13

- Zsigmondy/ Palmer system - 5│5

- FDI system –15 and 25

FUNCTIONS

- Premolars assist canines in tearing and cutting the food into smaller pieces.
- Premolars together with the molars help in maintaining the vertical length of the face.

DETAILED DESCRIPTION FROM ALL ASPECTS

BUCCAL ASPECT

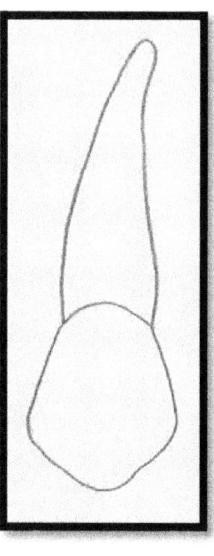

- The crown has a trapezoidal shape, with the shortest uneven side positioned cervically and the longest uneven side located occlusally.
- The mesial outline has a small concavity from the cervical line to the mesial contact area, situated in the central portion of the middle third of the crown.
- The distal outline is linear from the cervical line to the distal contact area. The distal contact region is wider than the mesial side. It is located near the junction of the middle and occlusal thirds.
- The buccal cusp is shorter and less pointed than that of the first premolar. The mesial slope of the cusp is shorter, whereas the distal slope is longer. The buccal cusp tip is positioned mesial to the line that bisects the buccal surface of the crown.
- The buccal surface of the crown is convex, having a well-defined buccal ridge.

It extends from the cusp tip to the cervical line. Shallow depressions are observed on both sides of this ridge.
- The root is conical, elongated, narrow and terminates in a blunt apex. The apical part of the root has a distal curve.

PALATAL ASPECT
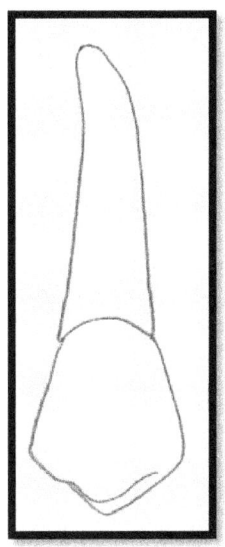
- The crown and the root narrows towards the palate. Consequently, parts of the mesial and distal surfaces of the crown and root are observable from this aspect.
- Palatal cusp is narrower mesiodistally compared to the buccal cusp. The cusp is smooth and spheroidal. Cusp tip is pointed with the mesial and distal slopes joining at right angle. Sometimes *'lingual ridge'* may also be seen on the palatal cusp running from the cusp tip to the cervical line.
- The palatal cusp is equivalent in length to the buccal cusp. The mesial and distal curves of the crown are convex and continue with the mesial and distal inclines of the palatal cusp.
- The palatal surface of the root is smooth and convex.
- <u>Root</u> -- It gradually narrows from the cervical line and concludes with a blunt apex.

MESIAL ASPECT
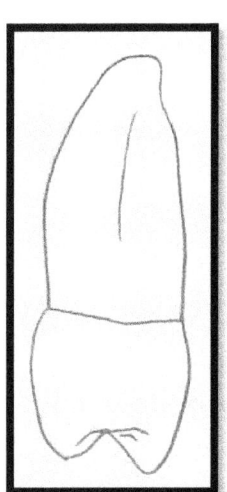
- From the mesial perspective, the crown exhibits the distinctive shape of posterior teeth, characterized as trapezoidal, with the smallest uneven side arranged occlusally and the longest uneven side positioned cervically.
- A defining property of all posterior maxillary teeth is that the cusp tips are situated well within the confines of the root trunk.
- The buccal and lingual curves of the crown are smooth and convex from the cervical line to the cusp tip.
- Crest of curvature buccally is located at the junction of the cervical and middle thirds, whereas palatally, it is situated at the midpoint of the middle third.
- Both cusps are visible from this perspective and are of identical height.
- The mesial marginal ridge is located at the intersection of the middle and occlusal thirds.
- The cervical line is less pronounced and oriented occlusally.
- It possesses a single root that manifests as a tapering cone. Developmental depression is observed on the root.
- In contrast to the first premolar, there is an absence of a developmental depression on the mesial surface of the crown (i.e., canine fossa) and no developmental groove crosses the mesial marginal ridge.

DISTAL ASPECT

- With a few exceptions, the distal and mesial aspects have been almost identical.
- Compared to the mesial side, there is a deeper developmental depression over the root.

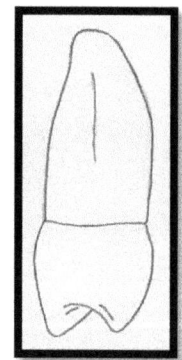

OCCLUSAL ASPECT

- The buccal surface is more noticeable compared to lingual surface from this aspect.
- This crown shows buccolingual tapering.
- The occlusal table is more ovoid or rounder. Mesiobuccal, distobuccal, mesiopalatal, distopalatal, mesial, and distal are the six sides.
- Every maxillary posterior tooth has a broader crown buccolingually than mesiodistally.
- Mesial and distal contact areas appear to be at the same level.
- Both marginal ridges and cusp ridges surround the occlusal table.

Cusp ridges – There are four of these. Mesiobuccal, distobuccal, distopalatal, and mesiopalatal. Mesiobuccal cusp ridge of the buccal cusp forms an acute angle with the mesial marginal ridge.

Triangular ridges – The triangle ridges are named after the cusps on which they are found and are two in number. On the buccal cusp, *buccal triangular ridge* runs from the central groove to the cusp tip. Similarly *lingual triangular ridge* traverses from the central groove to the tip of the lingual cusp.

Transverse ridge – The two triangular ridges of the buccal and palatal cusps join to form the transverse ridge in the center of the occlusal surface.

Marginal ridges – Of the two marginal ridges, (mesial and distal marginal ridges) mesial one is shorter. As opposed to the first premolar, the mesial marginal ridge is not crossed by any groove.

Grooves – The occlusal surface exhibits a wrinkled appearance owing to the presence of several additional grooves radiating from the center groove. The central developmental groove is short and uneven. It divides the occlusal surface in a buccolingual orientation. It traverses the inferior region of the central fossa on the occlusal surface, extending from the mesial pit to the distal pit. Two collateral grooves merge with this groove immediately within the mesial and distal marginal ridges. These are referred to as the *mesiobuccal developmental groove* and the *distobuccal developmental groove*. At the junction of these grooves with the central groove, there exist deep pits known as mesial and distal developmental pits.

Fossae -- The triangular depression known as the mesial triangular fossa, which contains the mesiobuccal development groove, is located just distal to the mesial marginal ridge. The triangular depression known as the distal triangular fossa, which contains the distobuccal development groove, is located just mesial to the distal marginal ridge.

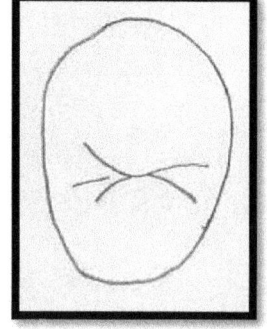

FIRST MOLAR
MAIN QUESTION

Q1) Describe the morphological aspects of permanent maxillary first molar.

Answer –

INTRODUCTION

- First molars are positioned in front of the permanent maxillary second molars and distal to the second premolars.
- It is the maxillary arch's largest tooth.

FUNCTIONS

a) They aid in food grinding and play a significant part in mastication.
b) They preserve the face's vertical dimension.
c) They maintain the continuity and integrity of dental arches.
d) They help to maintain esthetics by keeping the cheeks full.

TOOTH NOTATION

- Universal system – 3 and 14
- Zsigmondy/ Palmer system – 6 | 6
- FDI system –16 and 26

DETAILED DESCRIPTION FROM ALL ASPECTS

BUCCAL ASPECT

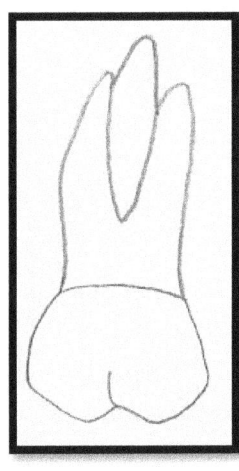

- The occlusal surface is the longest irregular side and the cervix the shortest of the trapezoidal form of the crown.
- Generally, the outline shape is straight from the cervical line to the point of contact in the mesial region. This outline descends distally before joining the mesial slope on the mesiobuccal cusp.
- Starting with the cervical line, the distal outline is convex until it joins the distobuccal cusp.
- Mesially the contact area is situated at the meeting point of occlusal and middle thirds. Whereas on the distal side it is in center of middle third of the crown.
- Each of the four cusps is partially visible from the buccal aspect.

- Mesiobuccal cusp seems to be wider than the distobuccal cusp. Cusp slopes (mesial and distal) of the mesiobuccal cusp contact at obtuse angle while that of distobuccal cusp is perpendicular, making this cusp more pointed. Height of both cusps is same.
- The two buccal cusps are separated by the buccal groove, which terminates almost at the middle third of the buccal surface on the crown. Typically, this groove ends in the buccal pit.
- With the convexity pointing towards the root, the cervical line exhibits very little curvature.
- There are three roots on the tooth: palatal, distobuccal, and mesiobuccal. All are visible from the buccal aspect. They are all derived from the same root trunk.
- The distance between trifurcation and cervical line is nearly 4 mm.
- The mesiobuccal root takes a straight course from the cervical line and in its middle third it curves distally.
- Beginning at the bifurcation, the root trunk exhibits a deep developmental groove.

PALATAL ASPECT

- Two lingual cusps and an additional cusp are noticeable from the palatal side. The tooth's longest and largest cusp is the mesiopalatal cusp. Its mesial and distal slopes meet at a specific obtuse angle.
- The distolingual cusp has a spheroidal form and is smooth. Cusp slopes do not form an angle.
- An accessory fifth cusp, the cusp of Carabelli, is located on the palatal surface of the mesiopalatal cusp. It is situated approximately 2 mm cervically from the cusp ridges of the mesiopalatal cusp.
- The palatal groove divides the two palatal cusps.
- From this angle, only the palatal root is visible. Parts of mesiobuccal and the distobuccal roots can be seen in the background. The palatal root has a blunt apex and is conical.

MESIAL ASPECT

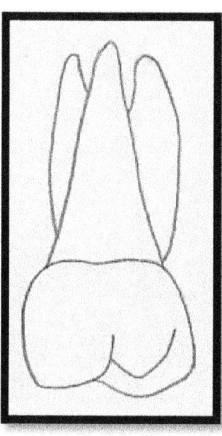

- The basic morphology of each of the posterior teeth is trapezoidal. The cervix is the longest uneven side and the occlusal region the shortest.
- The buccal contour is convex that extends from the cervical line to the crest of curvature, located in the center of the cervical third of the crown.
- The palatal outline of the crown is convex when the cusp of Carabelli is improperly developed.
- The mesial marginal ridge is clearly well-formed. It is longer buccolingually and is more occlusal compared to the distal marginal ridge.
- Cervical line -- irregular and directed occlusally.
- Both palatal and mesiobuccal roots can be viewed, of which the latter is broad with blunt tip.
- Palatal root is thinner, longer with pointed apex.

DISTAL ASPECT

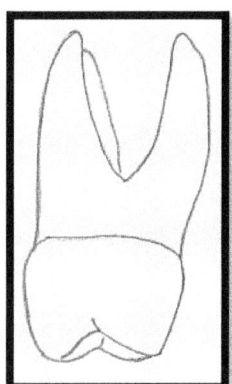

- With a few exceptions, the crown and root morphology resembles as that on the mesial side.
    a) Major portion of the buccal surface may be observed from this perspective since the crown's buccal surface tapers distally. As a result, the crown's buccolingual measurement mesially is larger than its distal measurement.
    b) In contrast to the mesial marginal ridge the distal marginal ridge is more cervically orientated.
    c) Cervical line runs nearly straight course.

OCCLUSAL ASPECT

- The crown seems roughly rhomboidal when viewed from this perspective.
- The buccolingual measurement is larger than the mesiodistal measurement.
- Mesiodistal tapering of the crown gives the impression that the mesial side of the crown is wider than the distal.
- The crown's palatal side seems wider than its buccal side.

Cusps

- One accessory cusp (the Carabelli cusp) and four major cusps are visible.
- Decreasing order of size -- mesiopalatal, mesiobuccal, distopalatal, distobuccal, cusp of Carabelli.

Ridges

- There are three visible ridges.

Oblique ridge – The occlusal surface is crossed obliquely by a ridge. It is created when the mesiopalatal cusps and the distobuccal cusp's triangular ridges unite. Often a groove partially or totally crosses the oblique ridge.

Marginal ridges – Mesial marginal ridge is broader buccolingually compared to the distal marginal ridge.

Transverse ridge – It is not well defined. Triangular ridges of mesiobuccal cusp and mesiolingual cusps join to form this transverse ridge.

Fossae

- Two major along two minor fossae are present.

Major fossae – Central and distal fossae constitute major fossae.

Minor fossae – Mesial and distal triangular fossae comprise of minor fossae

- *Central fossa* – Its shape is triangular. There is a central pit in the middle of this fossa.
- *Distal fossa* – It is situated behind the oblique ridge. Distal oblique groove is found at its base.
- *Triangular fossae* – The mesial triangular fossa is located distal to the mesial marginal ridge whereas the distal triangular fossa is present mesial to the distal marginal ridge.

Grooves

- Six grooves present. They're…….
- **Central developmental groove** – It arises at the central pit located in the central fossa. From there it traverses forward towards the mesial triangular fossa, and before ending it gives rise to two supplemental grooves.

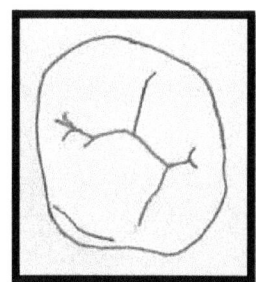

Buccal developmental groove– This also starts in the central pit and extends inbetween the two buccal cusps before ending on the buccal surface.

Distal oblique groove– It arises in the distal fossa, traverses posteriorly to end in the distal triangular fossa. Before fading, it gives two additional grooves.

Palatal developmental groove – The distal oblique groove which started in the distal fossa runs beyond each of the palatal cusps and ends on the palatal surface. It is referred to as the palatal developing groove.

Transverse groove of oblique ridge – It is a shallow groove which arises from the central developmental groove and typically disappears before it reaches the oblique ridge's crest. However it occasionally crosses it to join the distal oblique groove in the distal fossa.

Fifth cusp groove – This is present only in first molars. It is situated on the mesiopalatal cusp and gives outline to the fifth cusp. Finally it meets the palatal groove present between the two palatal cusps.

SECOND MOLAR

MAIN QUESTION

Q1) Describe the morphological aspects of permanent maxillary second molar.

Answer –

INTRODUCTION

- Maxillary second molars are one each on either side of the arch.
- They are located anterior to the third molar and posterior to the first molar.

FUNCTIONS

- It supplements the first molar in its function.
- It assists in grinding of food.

- They preserve the face's vertical dimension.
- They help to maintain the integrity of dental arches.
- They help to maintain the esthetics by keeping the cheeks full.

TOOTH NOTATION

- Universal system – 2 and 15
- Zsigmondy/ Palmer system – 7│7
- FDI system –17 and 27

DETAILED DESCRIPTION FROM ALL ASPECTS

BUCCAL ASPECT

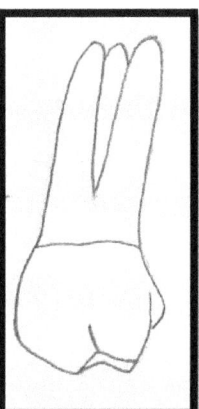

- The cervix region is the shortest uneven side and the occlusal side the longest of the crowns trapezoidal shape.
- In comparison to the maxillary first molar, the crown is narrower mesiodistally and considerably shorter cervico-occlusally.
- Mesial border is straight above the cervical line till the contact area. From here it turns distally and continues with the mesial slope of the mesiobuccal cusp.
- Distal outine of crown appears more convex above the cervical line till it continues with the distal slope of the distobuccal cusp.
- At the junction of occlusal and middle third of the crown, lies the mesial contact area. Whereas that on the distal side is in the center of middle third.
- Small portion of all the cusps can be seen from this aspect.
- Distobuccal cusp is smaller and mesiodistally narrower than the mesiobuccalcusp. Mesiobuccalcusp's mesial and distal slopes join at obtuse angle unlike the distobuccal cusp's, which meet at right angle.
- The two buccal cusps are set apart by the buccal developmental groove, which ends nearly in the middle of the buccal surface.
- The cervical line shows very little curvature, with the convexity orientated towards the root.
- Three roots noticeable from this aspect are palatal, distobuccal, and mesiobuccal. All of them originate from the same root trunk. The distance between both cervical line and the trifurcation point is approximately 4 mm.
- A deep developmental groove that begins at the bifurcation is visible on the root trunk.

PALATAL ASPECT

- The palatal side shows the two lingual cusps. The tooth's longest and largest cusp is the mesiopalatal cusp. An obtuse angle is formed at the junction of its distal and mesial slopes.
- The distolingual cusp has a spheroidal form and is smooth.
- The palatal groove separates the two palatal cusps.
- From this angle, only the palatal root is visible. It is in line with the tip of the distolingual cusp and has a conical, blunt apex.

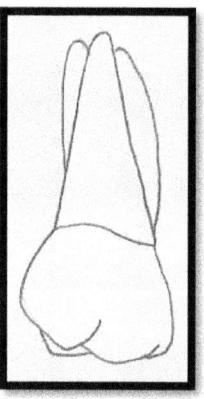

MESIAL ASPECT

- The posterior teeth's basic shape is trapezoidal. The longest uneven side is found on the cervix, while the occlusal table provides the shortest uneven side.
- Mesial marginal ridge is well formed. It is buccolingually wider and positioned more occlusal than the marginal ridge at the distal end.
- This cervical line is directed occlusally and is irregular.
- The palatal and mesiobuccal roots are visible from this perspective. Its mesiobuccal root is broader buccolingually and has a blunt apex. The palatal root has sharp apex and is thinner and longer.
- The roots are positioned within the buccolingual crown outline.

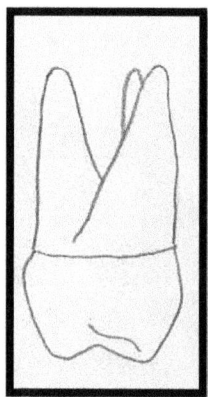

DISTAL ASPECT

- With a few exceptions, the distal and mesial aspects are comparable.
a) Mesiobuccal cusp is more visible from this side due to smaller dimension of the distobuccal cusp.
b) Mesiolingual cusp is unseen from this aspect.
c) The palatal root's apex and the distolingual cusp are in same line.
d) The distal marginal ridge has a shorter buccolingual length and is positioned higher cervically than the mesial marginal ridge.
e) Due to distal tapering of the buccal side of crown, the buccolingual width on the mesial side is more than that on distal.

OCCLUSAL ASPECT

Maxillary second molar shows two forms in relation to the occlusal aspect.

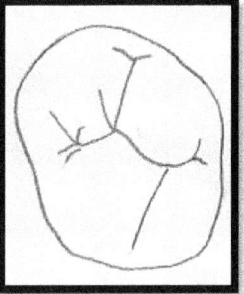

- *First type* -- Most of the teeth resemble the first molar.
- Buccolingual width is nearly identical to that of the first molar. However, the mesiodistal diameter is 1 mm short than first molar.
- The mesial side of the crown appears wider than the distal side due to mesiodistal tapering.
- The crown looks more slender on the palatal side than on the buccal due to buccolingual tapering.
- The mesiolingual and mesiobuccal cusps are just as big and fully formed like that of first molar. Distolingual and distobuccal cusps, however, are smaller.
- Supplemental grooves may also be seen.
- *Second type* -- This resembles third molar. Distolingual cusp development is inadequate. This gives a heart- shape form from the occlusal aspect.

****

Permanent Mandibular Teeth

CENTRAL INCISOR
MAIN QUESTION

Q1) Describe the morphological aspects of permanent mandibular central incisor.

Answer –

INTRODUCTION

- Two mandibular central incisors are placed on either side of imaginary midline.
- *Only the mandibular and maxillary central incisors have mesial surfaces that are touching with one another within the dental arches.*
- It is the dental arches' tiniest tooth.

TOOTH NOTATION

- Universal system – 24 and 25
- Zsigmondy/ Palmer system – 1 | 1
- FDI system – 31 and 41

DETAILED DESCRIPTION FROM ALL ASPECTS

LABIAL ASPECT

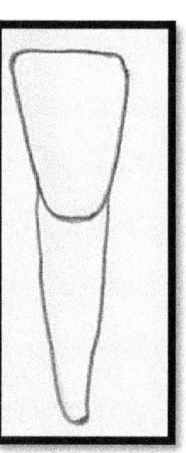

- From this field of vision, the crown has a trapezoidal shape with shortest uneven side cervically and largest incisally.
- The crown appears long and narrow due to its lesser mesiodistal width in comparison to the crown height.
- It has a smooth labial surface. It is convex in the cervical area and flat in the middle and incisal thirds.
- Incisal ridge is straight and positioned at right angle to the line that bisects the crown and root.
- From the sharp mesial and distal incisal angles, the crown tapers smoothly down to the root apex.
- Both the mesial and distal contact zones are on the same level i.e., at the junction of the incisal and middle thirds (characteristic feature).
- The cervicoincisal length of a crown on mesial and distal sides is the same.
- Cone-shaped root is narrower mesiodistally. The crown and root's mesial and distal contour is in continuation. Distal tilt is seen at the apical third and its mesial and distal side's tapers uniformly across the cervical line towards the root apex.

LINGUAL ASPECT

- It has a smooth lingual surface. The shallow lingual fossa is surrounded by incisal and marginal ridges which are not prominent.
- Small, smooth, convex cingulum lies in the cervical third.
- Both the crown and the root taper on the lingual side. This tapering makes it possible to see the depressions present on the mesial and distal sides of the root.
- It appears that the root has an evenly tapering cone with a slight distal curve in the apical thirds.

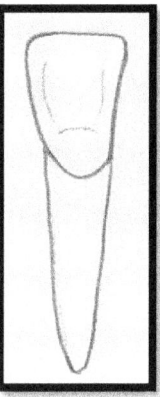

MESIAL ASPECT

- The crown has a trapezoidal form, the base of which is represented by the cervical line and the apex being at the incisal ridge.
- Crest of curvature both labially and lingually lies just above the cervical line.
- Crest of curvature on the labial side is at the cervical third. From here the surface descends straight and flat till the incisal ridge.
- The incisal ridge is positioned on the lingual side of the line that bisects the crown and root.
- Curvature of the cervical line is towards crown. This curvature is more on the mesial side than on the distal.
- The root is broad labiolingually. Its labial and lingual outlines remain almost parallel up to the middle third, after which they taper, terminating in either a blunt or pointed root apex.
- Developmental depression is seen on most of the root length.

DISTAL ASPECT

- The distal surface of the root or crown are comparable to that of mesial side.
- Curvature of the cervical line distally is lesser than on the mesial side.
- Developmental depression on root this side may be more marked.

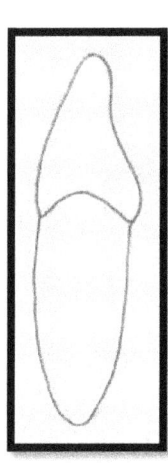

INCISAL ASPECT

- The crown has a triangular shape, with labial surface forming the base and the cingulum being the apex of the triangle when seen from the incisal aspect.
- The mesiodistal measurement is lesser than the labiolingual [opposite of maxillary anterior teeth].
- The crown appears bilaterally symmetrical.
- This aspect shows more of the labial surface due to the lingual inclination of the crown.
- The crown tapers labiolingually.
- *Very important unique feature among mandibular central and with lateral incisors could be noticed from the incisal aspect.* The incisal ridge of the central incisor aligns at right angle with the line bisecting the crown mesiodistally. Whereas the incisal ridge on the lateral incisor is not at right angle to this line, and hence it looks to be distolingually twisted. As a result, in lateral incisors, the distoincisal angle seems to be oriented lingual to the mesioincisal angle. This is to align with the shape of the dental arch.
- The labial surface appears flat despite some convexity in the cervical third.
- There is a little concavity on the lingual surface.

****

LATERAL INCISOR
MAIN QUESTION

Q1) Describe the morphological aspects of permanent mandibular lateral incisor.

Answer –

INTRODUCTION

- It is located anterior to the canine and distal to the central incisor.
- It very closely resembles mandibular central incisor.
- It has a little more size than the central incisor.

TOOTH NOTATION

- Universal system – 23 and 26
- Zsigmondy/ Palmer system – $\overline{2|2}$
- FDI system –32 and 42

DETAILED DESCRIPTION FROM ALL ASPECTS

LABIAL ASPECT

- The crown's shape appears trapezoidal with shortest uneven side cervically and largest incisally.
- The crown appears long and narrow due to lesser mesiodistal dimension in comparison to the crown height.
- The labial layer is smooth. At the cervical one-third it is convex, and rest in the middle third and incisal third its flat.
- Mesioincisal angle is sharp, and distoincisal angle is rounded.
- Even tapering of the mesial and distal sides till the root apex is noted.
- As the incisal ridge tapers by 1 mm from the mesial to the distal side, the mesial side's point of contact is higher than that of distal side.
- Mesiodistally, the root appears thin. Both root and crown's mesial and distal boundaries are continuous. It shows uniform narrowing starting from the cervical line to the apex of root. The root apex tapers distally and is pointed.

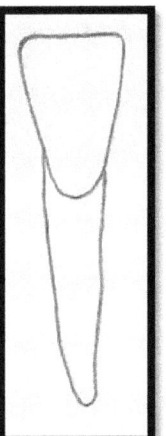

LINGUAL ASPECT

- The surface is smooth. All ridges (incisal, mesial and distal marginal ridges) are undeveloped and broad shallow lingual fossa is visible.
- The cingulum is small and smoothly convex.
- Lingually, the root and crown taper. This tapering makes it possible to see the development depression from this angle on both the mesial as well as distal sides of the root.
- The root looks like a cone that taper uniformly, with a slight distal curve in the apical third.

MESIAL ASPECT

- From this perspective, the crown has a triangular shape, with apex at the incisal ridge and base formed by the cervix.
- The distal sloping of the incisal ridge, gives an impression of mesial side of crown being longer than the distal side.
- Labial side surface of the crown above the crest of curvature which is located in cervical third is straight and flat. Later it slopes evenly till the incisal ridge.
- Crest of curvature labially and lingually is close to the cervical line.
- The incisal ridge is positioned on the lingual side of the line that bisects the crown and root.

- Curvature of the cervical line is towards crown. This curvature is more on the mesial side than on the distal.
- Compared to the central incisor, the root seems a little longer. It is labiolingually broad. Its lingual and labial outlines are almost parallel until the middle third after which it tapers to end in a blunt or a pointed root apex.
- There is developmental depression along much of the root's length.

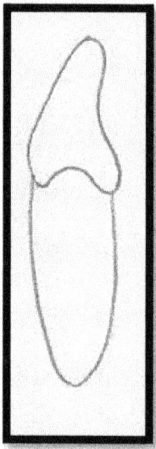

DISTAL ASPECT

- The distal side of both the root and crown is similar to the mesial side.
- The cervical line curves less than the mesial side.
- Root's developmental depression could be more pronounced.

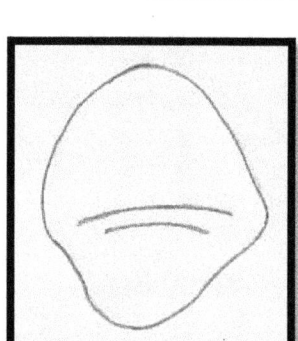

INCISAL ASPECT

- When seen from the crown's incisal aspect, it is essentially triangular in morphology, with the base created by the labial face and the apex pointing towards the cingulum.
- The labiolingual breadth is greater than the crown's mesiodistal breadth [this is opposite of maxillary anterior teeth].
- Due to labiolingual tapering of the crown, there is greater surface area on the labial side than on the lingual.
- *Very important unique feature among mandibular central and with lateral incisors could be noticed from the incisal aspect.* The incisal ridge of the central incisor aligns at right angle with the line bisecting the crown mesiodistally. Whereas the incisal ridge on the lateral incisor is not at right angle to this line, and hence it looks to be distolingually twisted. As a result, in lateral incisors, the distoincisal angle seems to be oriented lingual to the mesioincisal angle. This is to align with the shape of the dental arch.
- The labial surface appears flat with some convexity at the cervical third.
- The lingual surface has a little concavity.

CANINE
MAIN QUESTION

Q1) Describe the morphological aspects of permanent mandibular canine.

Answer –

INTRODUCTION

- Mandibular canines are two in number, one each on right and left sides.
- Mesially it has lateral incisor and distally the first premolar.
- Bifurcated roots may also be found.

FUNCTIONS

Functionally these are similar to the maxillary canines

- ✓ Supports lips and facial musculature.
- ✓ Assists in cutting and tearing food.
- ✓ Guides occlusion.
- ✓ Act as excellent abutments for fixed or removable prosthesis.

TOOTH NOTATION

- Universal system – 22 and 27
- Zsigmondy/ Palmer system – ⌐3 | 3⌐
- FDI system – 33 and 43

DETAILED DESCRIPTION FROM ALL ASPECTS

LABIAL ASPECT

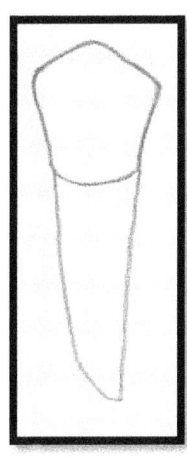

- The crown is trapezoidal in shape.
- Because the root and crown are mesiodistally thin, the cervicoincisal length appears more than maxillary canine.
- *Cervical line* – It shows uniform convexity which is directed towards the root apex.
- Labial surface is smooth. The labial ridge is less prominent than the maxillary canine. This ridge traverses in the center of the crown in a cervicoincisal direction. A line drawn across the ridge's crest is tilted slightly mesially.
- The root and the crown's mesial outlines are nearly straight and continuous. The mesioincisal angle and the mesial contact region are closer together.

- The mesial contact area is higher than the distal contact area.
- This cusp has distal and mesial ridges. The mesial cusp ridge is shorter than the distal. The cusp tip is positioned mesially relative to the line that divides the crown and root.
- The root is long, slender, and conical, with mesial and distal outlines that smoothly taper to a blunt or pointed apex. Occassionally, the apical third may show a mesial or distal curvature.

LINGUAL ASPECT

- The form of the crown is trapezoidal.
- Both crown and root shows lingual tapering.
- Cingulum is less bulky.
- Above the cingulum there is shallow less noticeable mesial and distal marginal ridges that encompass the entire lingual fossa the surface which appears smooth.
- In contrast to the distal marginal ridge, the mesial marginal ridge is longer and straighter.
- Cervical line is directed apically and is more curved.
- Because of lingual taper, much of the roots mesial and distal surfaces, as well as the developmental depressions they have on root can be noted.

MESIAL ASPECT

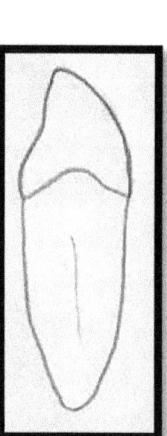

- The crown seems to be trapezoidal shaped from this angle.
- Compared to maxillary canines, the labial contour is less convex. In the cervical third, the crest of curvature is placed and is closer to the cervical line.
- Lingual outline also presents lesser convexity and concavity between the cervical line from the cusp tip due to presence of shallow lingual fossa and a poorly formed cingulum. On the lingual side the curvature's crest is in cervical third.
- Cusp tip looks much thinner due to less bulk of labial and lingual ridges.
- Due to lingual inclination of the crown, the cusp tip appears to be positioned on the lingual side of the line that bisects the crown and root.
- Cervical line curves incisally.
- Labial and lingual root outlines are almost parallel till the middle third after which they taper sharply apically.
- Root surface shows developmental depression.

DISTAL ASPECT

- Apart from a few minor variations, it is comparable to what was seen on the mesial side.
- Cervical line curve is lesser on this side.
- The root depression is more pronounced than on the mesial side.

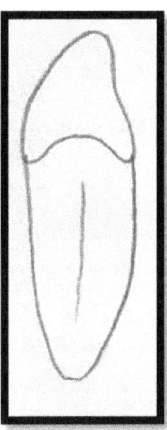

INCISAL ASPECT

- The outline of the crown is rhomboidal.
- The labiolingual dimension of the crown is larger than the mesiodistal dimension.
- Lingual tapering of the crown permits more visibility of the labial surface.
- The tip of the cusp is present on the lingual side of the line that splits the crown labiolingually.
- On the labial surface, the labial ridge is clearly visible.
- The mesial cusp slope is slightly labial to the distal cusp slope. Furthermore, the distoincisal angle is considerably lingual with respect to the mesioincisal angle. Because of this feature, the crown has a lingual twist.
- There is shallow lingual fossa, marginal ridges, and less noticeable cingulum on the lingual surface.

****

FIRST PREMOLAR
MAIN QUESTION

Q1) Describe the morphological aspects of permanent mandibular first premolar.

Answer –

INTRODUCTION

- The mandibular first premolars are located one each on the left and right sides.
- In contrast to the maxillary arch, the first premolar is typically smaller then the second.
- It lies posterior to canine and anterior to the second premolar. Hence it has characteristics resembling both canine and second premolar.

FUNCTIONS

- They assist canines in tearing and cutting the food into smaller pieces.
- Together with the molars, they also assist in preserving the face's vertical dimension.

TOOTH NOTATION

- Universal system – 21 and 28

- Zsigmondy/ Palmer system –

  $$\frac{}{4\,|\,4}$$

- FDI system – 34 and 44

DETAILED DESCRIPTION FROM ALL ASPECTS

BUCCAL ASPECT

- The structure is trapezoidal, featuring a shorter, irregular side at the cervical end and broader, uneven side at the occlusal end.
- Crown appears bilaterally symmetrical.
- The well-developed buccal lobe contributes to the formation of the buccal cusp.
- Starting at the cervical line, the mesial outline runs straight or slightly concave. It turns convex as it approaches the mesial contact area.
- Similarly, from the cervical line, the distal side takes a concave outline and becomes convex at the distal contact region.
- Contact area on both mesial and distal sides are at the same level i.e., at the center of the middle third of the crown.

- The distal cusp ridge is concave and somewhat longer than the mesial cusp, which is shorter and straighter.
- The buccal cusp tip is oriented mesially, in relation to an imaginary midline dividing the crown mesiodistally.
- The buccal ridge extends between the cusp tip and the cervical line.
- Cervical line shows convexity facing apically.
- The root has a long, thin, conical form. Its distal and mesial outlines gently taper in apical direction to end in a blunt apex.

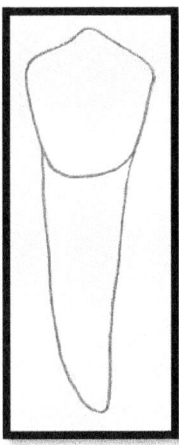

LINGUAL ASPECT

- Due to buccolingual tapering, one may observe both the root and crown's mesial and distal surfaces.
- Due to greater slope of the occlusal surface towards the lingual side, a larger portion of it is visible from this perspective.
- The lingual cusp appears undeveloped and is about half the height compared with the buccal cusp. It frequently has a pointed tip.
- A characteristic feature seen on the lingual surface of mandibular first premolar which also helps in differentiating from its adjacent second premolar is the presence of mesiolingual groove. This groove begins at the mesial fossa and ends on the lingual surface.
- Root evenly ends in a pointed apex after tapering from the cervical line.

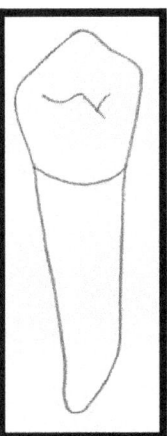

MESIAL ASPECT

- The crown form is rhomboidal.
- Root apex and buccal cusp tip are in same line.
- Prominent curvature of the buccal surface is noted starting from the cervical line to the buccal cusp tip. The crown's crest of curvature is situated where the middle and cervical thirds meet.
- The lingual outline is less curved than the buccal outline. The crest of curvature lying in the middle portion of the crown. The lingual cusp tip and lingual outline are placed in the same plane.
- There is lingual and cervical inclination of the mesial marginal ridge. It joins the mesiolingual groove at its termination.
- The cervical line is regular, occlusally inclined, and smooth.
- Labial and lingual root outlines taper gently from the cervical line and ends in pointed apex.
- Deep developmental depression is visible on the root's mesial surface.

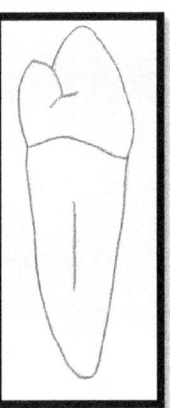

DISTAL ASPECT

- The distal and mesial aspects differ from one another.
- The distal marginal ridge is placed at a higher occlusal level than the mesial marginal ridge.
- The distal contact area is greater than the mesial. It is located in the center of the crown, midway between the cervical line, and the buccal cusp tip, and the lingual and buccal crown outlines.
- Less curvature is shown by the cervical line distally, when compared to the mesial aspect.
- Root exhibits shallow developmental depression than on mesial side.

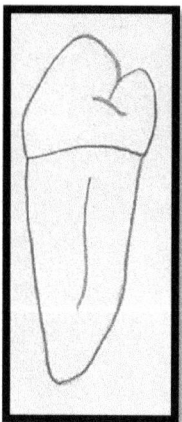

OCCLUSAL ASPECT

- In most teeth, occlusal outline is diamond shape.
- There is prominent buccal ridge on the buccal surface.
- The tip of the buccal cusp is located above the line that labiolingually divides the crown.
- Compared to the distal contact area, the mesial contact area is smaller.
- The lingual tilt of the crown makes much of the buccal surface visible.
- It has a tiny lingual cusp.

Ridges

Marginal ridge – There are two, the mesial and distal marginal ridges which are well-developed.

Fossae – The mesial and distal fossae are the two fossae. It is not known as triangular fossa because of its irregular shape. Within the mesial and distal marginal ridges, the distal and mesial fossae respectively are situated.

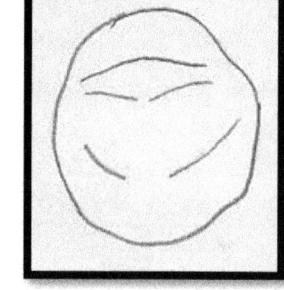

Pits: The distal fossa possesses a pit. Many additional grooves radiate from this pit.

Grooves

a) *Mesial developmental groove* – this short groove runs buccolingually in the mesial fossa.

b) *Mesiolingual developmental groove* – this groove starts from the mesial fossa and runs briefly on the mesiolingual surface. It is a characteristic feature found on mandibular first premolar.

c) *Distal developmental groove* – this long, crescent shaped groove is present in the distal fossa.

****

SECOND PREMOLAR
MAIN QUESTION

Q1) Describe the morphological aspects of permanent mandibular second premolar.

Answer –

INTRODUCTION

- There are two, on either side of the dental arch.
- In contrast to the first premolar, the second one is bigger.

FUNCTIONS

- They assist canines in tearing and cutting the food into smaller pieces.
- They also help in preserving the face's vertical dimension.

TOOTH NOTATION

- Universal system – 20 and 29
- Zsigmondy/ Palmer system –

   |
  ---+---
  5 | 5

- FDI system –35 and 45

DETAILED DESCRIPTION FROM ALL ASPECTS

BUCCAL ASPECT

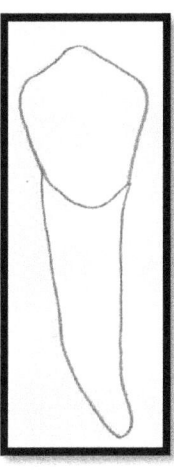

- It is trapezoidal, with the most significant uneven side occlusally, and the shortest uneven side cervically.
- The crown seems almost symmetrical on both sides.
- The well-developed middle buccal lobe forms a buccal cusp.
- The mesial outline being straight or slightly concave from cervical line becomes convex at the mesial contact area.
- The distal outline is convex at the distal contact area and concave above, till the cervical line.
- The contact region is vast and higher up mesially and distally.
- The buccal ridge runs between the buccal cusp tip and cervical line.
- The cervical line has minimal curvature with convexity facing apically.
- Root is conical in shape, long and broader mesiodistally. Its mesial and distal outlines gently taper in apical direction to end in a blunt apex.

LINGUAL ASPECT

- As in first premolar, the crown and root taper lingually, but comparatively to a lesser extent. As a result, this aspect shows minimal mesial with distal surfaces.
- Cusp or cusps are formed from the lingual lobe.
- Only a portion of the occlusal surface is visible from this view since the lingual cusp is as long as the buccal cusp.
- ***Three cusp type*** – in this type, the length and width of the mesiolingual cusp is greater, whereas the distolingual cusp is shorter and smaller. A lingual groove that extends a short distance along the lingual surface divides these cusps.
- ***Two-cusp type***–in this type, single large and long lingual cusp can be seen.
- Root evenly tapers to a pointed apex from the cervical line.

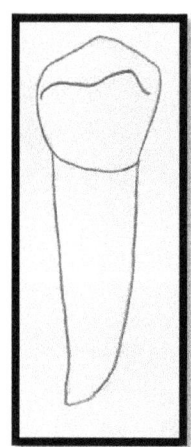

MESIAL ASPECT

- The crown outline has a rhomboidal shape.
- Buccolingually, both root and crown are broader.
- Compared to the first premolar, the buccal cusp is shorter.
- The buccal outline exhibits a remarkable curvature from the cervical line to the tip of the buccal cusp. The crest of curvature being at the intersection of the cervical and the middle third of the crown.
- The long axis of the tooth is perpendicular to the mesial marginal ridge.
- The occlusal curve of the cervical line is regular and smooth.
- Root tapers finely from the cervical line till the blunt apex. Root is longer.
- Deep developmental depression is visible on the root's mesial surface.

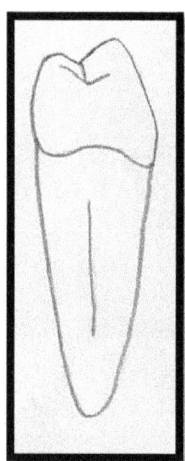

DISTAL ASPECT

- Distal aspect and the mesial side are nearly identical.
- Since the distal marginal ridge is lower, more of the occlusal surface is visible from this side.
- The crown exhibits mesiodistal tapering, just like every other posterior tooth.
- Compared to the mesial contact area, distal contact area is wider. It is situated midway between the buccal and lingual borders and between the cervical line and the tip of the buccal cusp.
- Compared to the mesial, the distal cervical line exhibits less curvature.
- Root exhibits shallow developmental depression than on mesial side.

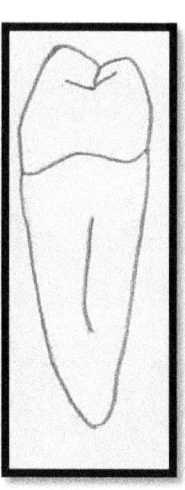

OCCLUSAL ASPECT

- The crown's lingual tilt allows most of the buccal surface to be observed from the occlusal perspective.
- Second premolar shows two forms: three-cusp type (more common) and two-cusp type.

Three-cusp type – It appears square shape. Three cusps are present: the largest is the buccal cusp, followed by mesiolingual cusp then the smallest, the distolingual cusp. Triangular ridges are highly formed on each cusp. Grooves divide the three cusps. Converging at the central pit, these grooves create a Y-shaped pattern on the occlusal table. Running from the central pit in a mesiobuccal direction, the long *mesial developmental groove* terminates at the mesial fossa which is present distal to the mesial marginal ridge. The shorter *distal developmental groove* runs from the central pit in a distobuccal direction to terminate at the distal fossa which is present mesial to the distal marginal ridge. In contrast to the distolingual cusp, the mesiolingual cusp is significantly wider mesiodistally. The lingual developmental groove separates the mesiolingual and distolingual cusps. It traverses from the central pit on the occlusal table, to end on the lingual surface.

- ***Two-cusp type*** – It appears round shape. The two cusps present are the buccal and lingual. Groove separating the buccal and lingual cusps is *central developmental groove*. It has a mesiodistal course and can be either crescent or straight. It ends in the *mesial and distal fossae. Additional grooves* are occasionally observed extending outward from the central groove. In the mesial and distal fossae, certain teeth may have *mesial and distal pits respectively.*

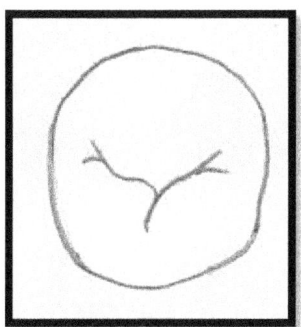

****

FIRST MOLAR
MAIN QUESTION

Q1) Describe the morphological aspects of permanent mandibular first molar.

Answer –

INTRODUCTION

- Mandibular first molars are the largest teeth in the lower arch.
- They are two in number, one on either side of the arch.
- They are distal to the second premolar and mesial to the second molar.
  FUNCTIONS

- They help in breaking the food into smaller particles.
- Guides occlusion.
- Provides vertical dimension of occlusion.

TOOTH NOTATION

- Universal system – 19 and 30
- Zsigmondy- Palmer system – ⌐⌐
  6 | 6

- FDI system –36 and 46

DETAILED DESCRIPTION FROM ALL ASPECTS

BUCCAL ASPECT

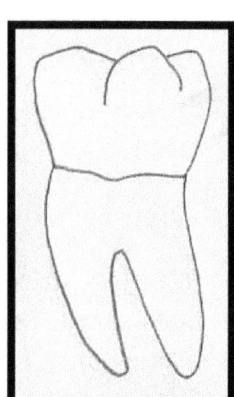

- From this aspect the crown is trapezoidal in shape with the uneven sides represented by the cervical and occlusal outlines.
- *Cusps* - All five cusps can be seen. The buccal cusps are in front and only the tips of the lingual cusps behind can be seen from this aspect. The three buccal cusps (mesiobuccal, distobuccal and distal) are nearly flat. Distal cusp is the smallest of the three and is slightly longer than the other two buccal cusps. Mesiobuccal cusp is flat and widest of all the buccal cusps.
- *Contact area* – mesially it is at the junction of the middle and the occlusal third and distally at the middle of middle third.
- *Grooves* – *Mesiobuccal developmental groove* separates the mesiobuccal and distobuccal cusp whereas the *distobuccal developmental groove* separates the distobuccal cusp and the distal cusp.
- *Cervical line* – It is regular and points towards the root.
- *Outline* – Mesial outline is concave from the cervical line and becomes convex at the contact area. The distal outline runs straight above the cervical line and becomes convex at the distal contact area.
- *Roots*– The two roots: mesial and distal can be seen from this aspect. Mesial root shows an initial curvature mesially from the cervical line till the middle portion. From here it curves distally to terminate in a blunt apex which is located below the mesiobuccal cusp. Bifurcation of the roots is nearly 3 mm below the cervical line. A developmental depression is seen on the root trunk.

LINGUAL ASPECT

- *Cusps* – Due to the convergence of the crown and root lingually (buccolingual tapering), part of the mesial and distal surfaces of crown and root can be seen from this aspect. From the lingual aspect three cusps are seen: two lingual cusps and the distal cusp. Lingual cusps are tall and pointed and hide the buccal cusps from view. Mesiolingual cusp is wider mesiodistally and its tip is slightly higher than the distolingual cusp.

- *Grooves* – Lingual developmental groove separates the two lingual cusps.
- *Contact area* – Mesial contact area is at a higher level than the distal.
- *Cervical line* – It is regular and points towards the root bifurcation.
- *Roots* – Due to the lingual convergence, mesial and distal surfaces of the root can be seen from this aspect. Root bifurcation is nearly 4 mm below the cervical line.

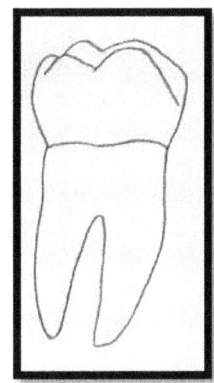

MESIAL ASPECT

- The crown has a rhomboidal outline. It shows lingual tilt which is characteristic of all mandibular posterior teeth.
- Buccolingual measurement of the crown and root is more mesially.
- Only the mesiobuccal cusp, mesiolingual cusp and mesial root are seen from this aspect.
- *Outline* – Buccal outline of crown is convex above the cervical line. Crest of curvature is at the cervical third. Lingual outline of crown runs from the cervical line in a lingual direction and becomes convex in the middle third of the crown. Crest of curvature lingually is in the middle of middle third of the crown.
- *Mesial marginal ridge* -- It is 1 mm below the cusp tips. It is confluent with the mesial ridges of the mesiobuccal and the mesiolingual cusps.
- *Cervical line* – Mesially the cervical line is irregular and curves occlusally or at times may run a straight course buccolingually.
- *Contact area* – mesially it is in the center between the buccal and lingual outlines.

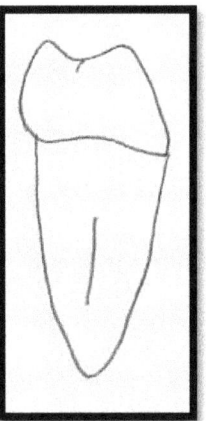

DISTAL ASPECT

- The crown has a rhomboidal outline.
- More of the tooth is seen from the distal aspect due to mesiodistal converging of the buccal and the lingual surfaces.
- More of the occlusal surface and some parts of all the five cusps can be seen.
- Distal contact area is at a higher level than the mesial contact area.
- Distal marginal ridge is short and is confluent with the cusp ridges of the distal and distolingual cusps.
- The distal root is narrower buccolingually.
- Cervical line runs a straight course buccolingually.

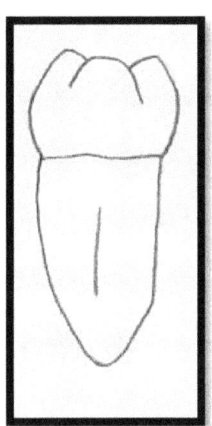

OCCLUSAL ASPECT

- The crown exhibits hexagonal outline.
- Mesiodistal width is 1mm more than the buccolingual width. Buccolingual width is more on the mesial side than on the distal and this is due to the mesiodistal tapering of the crown. Due to the buccolingual tapering of the crown the mesiodistal width on the buccal side is more than that on the lingual side.
- **_Cusps_** –Mesiobuccal cusp is slightly larger in size. The two lingual cusps are almost of similar size. The distobuccal cusp is smaller than these thee cusps. Distal cusp is the smallest of all the five cusps.
- **_Fossa_** – Occlusal surface of first molar shows one major fossa (*central fossa*) and two minor fossae (*mesial triangular fossa and distal triangular fossa*). Central fossa is present in the center of the occlusal surface between the buccal and the lingual cusps. Mesial triangular fossa is smaller than the central fossa and lies distal to the mesial marginal ridge. Distal triangular fossa is smaller than the mesial triangular fossa and lies mesial to the distal marginal ridge.
- **_Grooves_** – Numerous grooves are present on the occlusal surface. *Central developmental* groove runs in the center of the crown. It begins in the central pit located in the central fossa and runs an irregular course mesially and terminates at the mesial pit located in the mesial triangular fossa. *Mesiobuccal developmental* groove runs between the two buccal cusps and joins the central groove. From the central pit the central groove runs a short distance distobuccally and continues as *distobuccal developmental groove* between the distobuccal and distal cusps. *Lingual developmental groove* runs between the two lingual cusps. Sometimes *supplemental grooves* can also be seen.
- **_Pits_** – *Central pit* is present in the center of the central fossa. All the grooves converge in this pit. *Mesial pit* is present in the mesial triangular fossa.

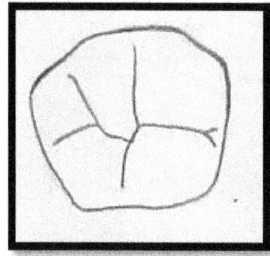

****

SECOND MOLAR
MAIN QUESTION

Q1) Describe the morphological aspects of permanent mandibular second molar.

Answer –

INTRODUCTION

- Mandibular second molars are two in number and are one on either side of the mandibular arch.
- It is distal to the first molar and mesial to the third molar.

FUNCTIONS

- It assists the first molar in breaking the food into smaller particles.
- Guides occlusion.
- Provides vertical dimension of occlusion.

TOOTH NOTATION

- Universal system – 18 and 31

- Zsigmondy/ Palmer system – 7 | 7

- FDI system –37 and 47

DETAILED DESCRIPTION FROM ALL ASPECTS

BUCCAL ASPECT

- From this aspect the crown is trapezoidal with the uneven sides represented by the cervical and occlusal surface.
- The crown is shorter cervico-occlusally and narrower mesiodistally when compared to the first molar.
- *Cusps* -- Only the mesiobuccal and the distobuccal cusps are seen from this aspect. These cusps have almost same mesiodistal dimension.
- *Grooves* – B*uccal developmental groove* separates the mesiobuccal and distobuccal cusps and runs for a short distance on the buccal surface.
- *Cervical line* – It is regular with apex pointing to the bifurcation.
- *Outline* – Mesial outline is concave from the cervical line and becomes convex at the contact area. The distal outline runs straight above the cervical line and becomes convex at the distal contact area.

- ***Roots*** – The two roots: mesial and distal can be seen from this aspect. They are shorter than those in first molar and are often closer together with their axes nearly parallel. Mesial root tip is located below the mesiobuccal cusp. Bifurcation of the roots is nearly 3 mm below the cervical line. Developmental depression is seen on the root trunk.

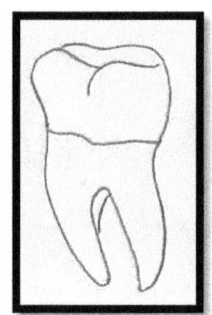

LINGUAL ASPECT

- ***Cusps*** – Due to the slight tapering of the crown and root lingually (buccolingual tapering), little of the mesial and distal surfaces of crown and root can be seen from this aspect. From the lingual aspect the two lingual cusps are seen.
- ***Grooves*** – *Lingual developmental groove* separates the two lingual cusps and runs a short distance on the lingual surface.
- ***Contact area*** – Mesial contact area is at a higher level than the distal contact area. When compared to the first molar the contact areas are at a lower level.
- ***Cervical line*** – It is irregular and points towards the root bifurcation.
- ***Roots*** – Root bifurcation is nearly 4 mm below the cervical line.

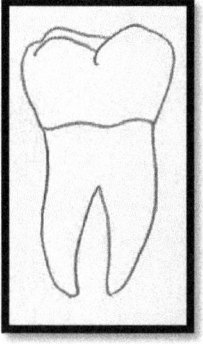

MESIAL ASPECT

- The crown has a rhomboidal outline. It shows lingual tilt which is characteristic of all mandibular posterior teeth.
- Buccolingual measurement of the crown and root is more mesially.
- The mesiobuccal cusp, mesiolingual cusp and mesial root are seen from the mesial aspect.
- Occlusal surface is constricted buccolingually.
- ***Outline*** – Buccal outline of crown is convex above the cervical line. Crest of curvature is at the cervical third. Lingual outline runs from the cervical line straight in a lingual direction and becomes convex in the middle third of the crown. Crest of curvature lingually is in the center of middle third of the crown.
- ***Mesial marginal ridge*** -- It is 1 mm below the cusp tips. It is confluent with the mesial ridges of the mesiobuccal and the mesiolingual cusps.
- ***Cervical line*** – Mesially the cervical line shows less curvature being straight and regular buccolingually.
- ***Contact area*** -- Mesial contact area is centered buccolingually.

DISTAL ASPECT

- The crown has a rhomboidal outline.
- More of the occlusal surface and some parts of all the four cusps can be seen from this aspect.
- Distal contact area is at a lower level than the mesial contact area. It is centered buccolingually.
- Distal marginal ridge is short and confluent with the cusp ridges of the distobuccal and distolingual cusps.
- The distal root is narrower buccolingually.
- Cervical line runs a straight course buccolingually.

OCCLUSAL ASPECT

- The crown exhibits rectangular outline.
- The distal outline of the crown resembles a semicircle when compared to the rectangular outline of the mesial side.
- Mesiodistal width is more than the buccolingual width. Buccolingual width is more on the mesial side than on the distal due to mesiodistal tapering of the crown. Due to the buccolingual tapering of the crown the mesiodistal width on the buccal side is more than that of the lingual side.
- *Cusps* – Four cusps can be seen. Mesiobuccal, mesiolingual, distobuccal and distolingual. The four cusps are nearly of same size.
- *Fossa* – Occlusal surface of first molar shows one major fossa (*central fossa*) and two minor fossae (*mesial triangular fossa and distal triangular fossa*). Central fossa is present in the center of the occlusal surface between the buccal and the lingual cusps. Mesial triangular fossa lies distal to the mesial marginal ridge and is smaller than the central fossa. Distal triangular fossa lies mesial to the distal marginal ridge and is smaller than the mesial triangular fossa.
- *Grooves* – Numerous grooves are present on the occlusal surface. *Central developmental* groove runs in the center of the crown. It begins in the central pit located in the central fossa and runs an irregular course mesially and terminates at the mesial pit located in the mesial triangular fossa. *Buccal developmental* groove runs between the two buccal cusps. *Lingual developmental groove* runs between the two lingual cusps. The buccal and the lingual developmental grooves meet at the central groove at right angle and divide the occlusal surface in four equal parts. *Supplemental grooves* can also be seen.

****

Differences Between Teeth

DIFFERENCES – MAXILLARY CENTRAL AND LATERAL INCISORS

ASPECT	CENTRAL INCISOR	LATERAL INCISOR
LABIAL	<ul><li>Larger mesiodistally</li><li>Wider cervically</li><li>Mesioincisal angle 90^0</li><li>Mesial contact area -- incisal third.</li><li>Distal contact -- Junction of incisal and middle third</li><li>Root appears as long as crown.</li><li>Root tapers evenly</li></ul>	<ul><li>Smaller</li><li>Narrower</li><li>More rounded and acute</li><li>Junction of incisal and middle third</li><li>Middle third.</li><li>Root longer and narrower.</li><li>Root curves distally.</li></ul>
PALATAL	<ul><li>Lingual fossa -- large & shallow</li><li>Distal marginal ridge -- straight, almost as long as mesial marginal ridge.</li><li>Lingual pit and groove is rare.</li></ul>	<ul><li>Small but deep.</li><li>Short and curved.</li><li>Very common.</li></ul>
PROXIMAL	<ul><li>Cervical line curvature is deep.</li><li>Deep concavity of lingual fossa.</li></ul>	<ul><li>Curvature is less deep.</li><li>Shallow concavity</li></ul>
INCISAL	<ul><li>Crown significantly larger mesiodistally.</li><li>Labial surface appears broadly convex.</li><li>Incisal ridge curves mesiodistally with distoincisal angle more towards the palatal side when compared to the mesioincisal angle.</li></ul>	<ul><li>Mesiodistal and labiolingual width of crown appears roughly same.</li><li>More rounded and convex labial outline.</li><li>Incisal ridge is short & straighter mesiodistally.</li></ul>

DIFFERENCES – MAXILLARY FIRST AND SECOND PREMOLARS

Answer –

FIRST PREMOLAR	SECOND PREMOLAR
BUCCAL ASPECT	
Buccal ridge is prominent	Not so prominent
Shallow depression is present on either side of buccal ridge	These depressions are absent
Buccal cusp is long and pointed	Buccal cusp is short and blunt
Mesial cusp slope longer than the distal cusp slope.	Mesial cusp slope shorter than the distal cusp slope.
Buccal cusp tip is placed distal to the line bisecting the crown mesiodistally.	Buccal cusp tip is placed mesial to the line bisecting the crown mesiodistally.
PALATAL ASPECT	
Palatal cusp is shorter than the buccal cusp by about 1mm.	Palatal cusp is almost as long as the buccal cusp.
Crown tapers palatally	Less palatal tapering of crown.
PROXIMAL ASPECT	
Cusp tips appear closer together	Cusp tips appear wider.
Two roots present (not always).	Single root is seen
Developmental groove crosses the mesial marginal ridge.	This feature is absent.
Mesial developmental depression or canine fossa present on the mesial surface.	This feature is absent.
Deep developmental depression present on mesial aspect of root.	Shallower depression present on mesial aspect of root
OCCLUSAL ASPECT	
Crown appears as an asymmetric hexagon	Crown looks as a symmetrical oval
Prominent palatal taper of crown	Not so prominent palatal taper
Buccal aspect shows one prominent buccal ridge	Buccal ridge not so prominent
Mesiobuccal cusp ridge meets mesial marginal ridge at right angle	Mesiobuccal cusp ridge meets mesial marginal ridge at obtuse angle
Distal contact area is more buccal when compared with the mesial contact area.	Both contact areas are at same level

Mesial marginal groove crosses the mesial marginal ridge.	No such feature is present.
Fewer supplemental grooves present	More supplemental grooves present. Crown appears more wrinkled

DIFFERENCES –MAXILLARY FIRST AND SECOND MOLARS

MAXILLARY FIRST MOLAR	**MAXILLARY SECOND MOLAR**
BUCCAL ASPECT	
Crown is taller occlusocervically	Crown is shorter
Crown is broader mesiodistally	Crown is narrower
Deeper buccal developmental groove usually ends in a buccal pit	Buccal developmental groove does not usually terminate in a pit
Roots are more or less straight	Roots are more distally inclined
Curvature of buccal roots can be seen	Less curved buccal roots
PALATAL ASPECT	
Cusp of Carabelli is present on the palatal aspect of mesiopalatal cusp	Cusp of Carabelli mostly absent.
Palatal root is more or less parallel to long axis of tooth	Palatal root more distally inclined
OCCLUSAL ASPECT	
Greater mesiodistal width on palatal side of the crown.	Due to palatal taper, mesiodistal width on palatal side is lesser
Transverse ridge is present	Transverse ridge is absent
Pronounced, well developed oblique ridge present	Less significant oblique ridge

DIFFERENCES – MANDIBULAR CENTRAL AND LATERAL INCISORS

CENTRAL INCISOR	LATERAL INCISOR
Smaller in overall dimension.	Larger in dimension.
Labial view a) Mesial and distal contact areas are located at more or less at the same level. b) The cervicoincisal length of crown on mesial and distal sides is same c) The incisal ridge appears to be at right angle to the line bisecting the crown mesiodistally.	a) Distal contact area is more cervically located than mesial contact area. b) Cervicoincisal length on the mesial side is more than that on the distal side. c) The incisal ridge appears to slope from mesial towards the distal side.
Incisal view The incisal ridge is at right angle to the line bisecting the crown mesiodistally.	The incisal ridge appears to be distolingually twisted and not at right angle to the line bisecting the crown mesiodistally.
Distoincisal angle is sharp.	Distoincisal angle is rounded.

DIFFERENCES – MAXILLARY AND MANDIBULAR CANINE

Sl. No.	Maxillary canine	Mandibular canine
1	Crown is wider mesiodistally	Crown is narrower mesiodistally
2	Crown is shorter in length in most cases.	Crown is longer in length by 0.5-1 mm.
3	Root is longer in length.	Root is slightly shorter in length by 1-2 mm.
4	Labiolingual diameter of crown and root is slightly more.	Labiolingual diameter of crown and root is comparatively less.
5	Lingual surface shows well formed lingual fossa.	Lingual fossa is shallow and lingual surface appears smooth and flat.
6	Cingulum is well developed.	Cingulum is poorly developed.
7	Marginal ridges are bulky.	Marginal ridges are less bulky.
8	Cusp is well developed.	Cusp is not well developed.
9	Cusp ridges are thicker labiolingually.	Cusp ridges are thinner labiolingually.
10	From the incisal aspect, the cusp tip appears to lie labial to the line bisecting the crown labiolingually.	Cusp tip lies lingual to the line bisecting the crown labiolingually.

11	*Labial view* -- Mesial contact area is at the junction of the middle and the incisal thirds.	Mesial contact area is near the mesioincisal angle.
12	*Labial view* -- Distal contact area is at the middle of the middle third.	Distal contact area is more towards the incisal aspect but below the mesial contact area.
13	Root has a bluntly pointed apex.	Root apex is sharply pointed.
14	Root curvature is often in distal direction.	Root curvature is often in mesial direction.
15	*Mesial aspect* -- a) The crown shows more curvature labially below the cervical line. b) Cervical line curves less towards the incisal portion	a) The crown shows less curvature labially above the cervical line. b) Cervical line curves more towards the incisal potion
16	*Incisal aspect* – a) The mesial and distal cusp ridges are in a straight line mesiodistally. b) Mesial and distal contact points are nearly in same line.	a) The distal cusp ridge appear lingual to the mesial cusp ridge. b) Distal contact point lies lingual to the mesial contact point.

DIFFERENCES –MANDIBULAR FIRST AND SECOND PREMOLARS

FIRST PREMOLAR	SECOND PREMOLAR
BUCCAL ASPECT	
Crown is taller	Shorter crown
Buccal cusp is pointed	Less pointed buccal cusp
Depression in occlusal one third on either side of buccal ridge	Buccal surface uniformly smooth
Prominent buccal ridge	Buccal ridge less prominent
Short root with sharp apex	Long root with blunt apex
LINGUAL ASPECT	
More buccolingual tapering of crown.	Less buccolingual tapering of crown.
Lingual cusp is short, almost half of buccal cusp	Lingual cusp is long but shorter than buccal cusp
Much of occlusal surface can be viewed	Less of occlusal surface can be seen
Mesial and distal root depressions can be	Only distal depression of root can be seen

viewed due to more buccolingual tapering.	
Mesiolingual developmental groove is present.	It is absent.
PROXIMAL ASPECT	
Entire crown appears to be tilted lingually	Lesser inclination of crown lingually.
Very short, non functional lingual cusp	Lingual cusp is longer but shorter than the buccal cusp.
Mesial marginal ridge lower than distal marginal ridge	Distal marginal ridge lower than mesial ridge
Mesial marginal ridge slopes lingually in cervical direction.	Mesial marginal ridge perpendicular to long axis of teeth
Much of occlusal surface can be seen	Less of occlusal surface can be seen
Developmental depression on root is present on both proximal aspects, but distal depression is deeper	No depression on mesial aspect of root, only a shallow depression on the distal side.
OCCLUSAL ASPECT	
Asymmetrical rhomboidal outline	Ovoid outline in two-cusp type and square outline in three-cusp type
Prominent lingual taper	Lingual taper much less
Mesial half of crown narrower buccolingually	Distal half narrower
Mesial and distal developmental grooves run buccolingually in the mesial and distal fossa respectively.	In two-cusp type central groove is present. In three- cusp type, mesial, distal and lingual developmental grooves are present.

DIFFERENCES – MAXILLARY AND MANDIBULAR PREMOLARS

Characteristics	Maxillary	Mandibular
Buccal ridge	More prominent	Less prominent
Buccal and lingual cusp height	Not much difference.	More difference in height
Lingual tilt of the crown	Crown aligned over the root	Crown tilts more lingually
Crown shape	Oval or rectangular	Square or round
Crown width	Wider buccolingually	Wider mesiodistally
Canine fossa	Present on first premolar	Absent
Mesial marginal groove	Present on first premolar	Absent
Cusps	Second premolar has two cusps	Second premolar has two or three cusps

DIFFERENCES – MANDIBULAR FIRST AND SECOND MOLARS

FIRST MOLAR	SECOND MOLAR
GENERAL	
Overall dimensions is greater	Smaller dimension than first molars
Five cusps are present	Four cusps are present
BUCCAL ASPECT	
Cervicoocclusal taper of crown is pronounced	Less taper cervicoocclusally
Crown appears to sit right on the roots	Crown appears slightly distally tipped on its roots
Contact areas are located more occlusally	Contact areas are located more cervically
Roots show a greater flare from bifurcation area	Roots appear much closer together
Root trunk is short	Long root trunk
PROXIMAL ASPECT	
Mesial root is quite broad buccolingually	Narrower buccolingual dimension of mesial root
Mesial root has a blunt apex	More pointed apex of the mesial root
OCCLUSAL ASPECT	

Crown outline appears as irregular hexagon	Crown outline appears rectangular
Pronounced lingual taper of the crown	Much less lingual taper
Central groove traverses the occlusal surface in an irregular fashion.	Central groove is straight
Four major grooves present which form an irregular pattern over the occlusal surface of the crown.	Three major grooves present which form a "+" shape over the occlusal surface of the crown.
Five cusps	Four cusps
All cusps are of unequal size	All cusps are nearly of same size

DIFFERENCES – MAXILLARY AND MANDIBULAR MOLARS

Characteristic	**Maxillary**	**Mandibular**
Crown width	Wider buccolingually than mesiodistally	Wider mesiodistally than buccolingually
Number of roots	3	2
Oblique ridge	Present	Absent
Occlusal aspect	Rhomboidal	Rectangular
Functional cusps	4	4 or 5
Cusp of Carebelli	Present	Absent
Buccal cusps	2	2 or 3
Cusps sharpness	Buccal cusps are sharp and lingual cusps are rounded	Buccal cusps are rounded and lingual cusps are sharp
Buccal groove	1	2
Root trunk	Longer	Shorter
Buccal cervical ridge	Present	Absent

****

Mastication & Deglutition

SHORT NOTES

Q1) Mastication.

Answer -- Mastication is defined as a process where the consumed food is crushed into small pieces and mixed with saliva to form a bolus which can be readily swallowed.

INTRODUCTION

- Food is initially "incised" or bitten into smaller fragments by vertical mandibular movements. This is followed by tearing and grinding of food by lateral movements of mandible.
- As the food is transported from anterior to posterior sections of the dental aches, it is progressively reduced in size and mixed with saliva to form bolus.
- Although major portion of mastication is done by the occluding surfaces of the maxillary and mandibular teeth, some part is also carried out by pressing of the tongue against the rugae of hard palate.
- Mastication is a repetitive sequence of jaw opening and closing in the vertical plane and is called the masticatory cycle.

MASTICATORY CYCLE

Each masticatory cycle / chewing cycle lasts for approximately 0.8 to 1.0 seconds. Each masticatory cycle is composed of three phases.

1. Jaw opening phase
2. Rapid jaw closing phase
3. Slow jaw closing phase

Jaw opening phase

- In this phase there is separation of teeth. This is due to the depression of the mandible which is brought about by the activity of mylohyoid, anterior belly of diagastric, and inferior head of lateral pterygoid muscle.
- After the jaw separation, the heads of the condyles on either sides move anteriorly down the anterior surface of glenoid fossae, thereby causing protrusion of the mandible.

Rapid jaw closing phase

- This phase begins when the jaw opening phase comes to an end.
- In this phase the teeth are brought together.
- This rapid closing phase is brought about by the contraction of the masseter, medial pterygoid and temporalis muscles and horizontal movement brought about by contraction of lower fibers of temporalis and the lateral pterygoid muscles.

Slow jaw closing phase

- The rapid jaw closing phase ends when resistance is felt between the teeth. Then the slow jaw closing phase starts resulting in tooth to tooth contact.

- When the upper and lower teeth contact, the path of mandibular closure is determined by sliding of mandibular teeth along the cuspal inclines of the maxillary teeth.

MUSCLES INVOLVED IN MASTICATION

Masseter

Actions –
  a) Helps elevated mandible to close the mouth.
  b) Superficial fibers cause protrusion of mandible.

Temporalis

Actions –
  a) It elevates the mandible to close the mouth.
  b) It retracts the mandible after protrusion.
  c) It helps in side to side grinding movement.

Medial pterygoid

Actions-
  a) It elevates the mandible.
  b) It helps to protrude the mandible.
  c) Side to side movement of the mandible as a part of grinding movements.

Lateral pterygoid

Actions-
  a) Depresses the mandible to open the mouth.
  b) Moves the mandible from side to side.
  c) Protrudes the mandible.

****

Q2) Deglutition

Q) Stages or Phases of deglutition.

Answer --Deglutition or swallowing refers to the movement of the food from the oral cavity into the stomach.

- It starts as a voluntary act, it soon becomes involuntary.
- Human beings swallow approximately 600 times every 24 hour.

PHASES OR STAGES OF DEGLUTITION

Deglutition occurs in three phases/stages.
  a) Oral phase.
  b) Pharyngeal phase.
  c) Oesophageal phase.

ORAL PHASE

- This first stage is voluntary.
- It comprises of two sub phases.

  a] Forming a bolus of masticated food &,

  b] Forcing it posteriorly inside the oral cavity.

- Bolus formed during mastication is placed between the depressed dorsal surface of tongue and hard palate.
- The pressure required to push the bolus posteriorly, is generated by bringing the teeth in centric occlusion and producing a lip seal by contraction of orbicularis oris muscle.
- Tongue is then raised against the palate and the bolus present on the tongue is emptied antero-posteriorly, thereby pushing the bolus towards the pharynx posteriorly.
- In the oral phase, the airway remains open with the soft palate contacting the posterior surface of tongue thus forming a posterior oral seal.

PHARYNGEAL PHASE

- This second stage is involuntary.
- In this phase the bolus of food is pushed from the pharynx into the oesophagus.
- Pharynx is a common passage for both air and food. It divides into larynx and oesophagus. Larynx which is a respiratory passage lies anterior to oesophagus which continues downwards as the gastrointestinal (GI) tract.
- Pharynx communicates with mouth, nose, larynx and oesophagus. During this stage of deglutition, the bolus from the pharynx can enter into any of these openings.
- Various movements make the bolus enter only into the oesophagus. The entrance of bolus into other openings are prevented by following actions
✓ Return of bolus back into the mouth is prevented by the position of the tongue against the soft palate.
✓ Return of bolus into the nasopharynx is prevented by elevation of soft palate along with its extension (i.e. uvula).
✓ The movement of bolus forward into the larynx is prevented by (i) forward and upward movement of the larynx, (ii) by backward movement of epiglottis to seal the opening of larynx and (iii) by temporary stoppage of breathing.
✓ Since the other three openings are closed, the bolus now it has to pass only through the oesophagus. Various movements help for the free movement of the bolus in the oesophagus. The whole process takes in 1-2 seconds: upward movement of larynx stretches the opening of oesophagus and hence upper 3-4 cm of oesophagus relaxes. At the same time peristaltic waves begin in the pharynx due to the contraction of pharyngeal muscles.

OESOPHAGEAL PHASE

- The third stage is involuntary. In this stage bolus enters the stomach through the oesophagus.
- Main function of the oesophagus is to transport the bolus from the pharynx to the stomach. Movements of the oesophagus which transports the bolus into the stomach are called peristaltic waves.
- Peristalsis means a wave of contraction followed by wave of relaxation of GI tract muscles in a direction away from mouth. These waves are initiated when the bolus reaches the oesophagus. By this type of movement, the bolus is pushed down along the GI tract (oesophagus) finally into the stomach.

****

Q3) Deglutition and its nervous control.

Answer -- Deglutition or swallowing refers to the movement of the food from the oral cavity into the stomach.

- Beginning of deglutition (oral phase) is a voluntary act but later becomes involuntary and is carried out by a reflex action called deglutition reflex. It occurs during the pharyngeal and oesophageal phase.
- *Stimulus* – when the bolus enters the oropharyngeal region, the receptors present in this region are stimulated.
- *Afferent fibers* – afferent impulses from these oropharyngeal receptors pass via glossopharyngeal nerve to the deglutition center located in the floor of the fourth ventricle of the medulla oblongata of brain.
- *Efferent fibers* – efferent impulses from the deglutition center pass through the glossopharyngeal and the vagus nerves and reach soft palate, pharynx and oesophagus. The glossopharyngeal nerve controls the pharyngeal stage of deglutition and the vagus nerve with the oesophageal stage.
- *Response* – in response to the efferent impulse, there is upward movement of the soft palate to close the nasopharynx and upward movement of the larynx to close the respiratory passage so that the bolus enters the oesophagus. Now peristalsis occurs in the oesophagus pushing the bolus into the stomach.

****

Q4) Muscles of mastication.

Answer -- *Muscles associated with mastication are four in number. They are*

- ✓ Masseter
- ✓ Temporalis
- ✓ Lateral pterygoid
- ✓ Medial pterygoid

MASSETER

- It is a thick quadrilateral muscle which covers the lateral surface of the ramus of the mandible. It has a superficial and deep portion.
- The superficial part arises from the anterior two-third of the inferior border of the zygomatic arch, runs downwards and backwards and to gets inserted into the lateral surface of the mandibular ramus.
- The deep part arises from the posterior one-third of the inferior border of zygomatic arch and also from medial surface of this arch, runs vertically downwards and gets inserted into the lateral surface of the ramus.
- *Actions* –

    a) Helps elevated mandible to close the mouth.
    b) Superficial fibers cause protrusion of mandible.

TEMPORALIS MUSCLE

- It is a large fan shaped muscle occupying space in the temporal fossa and connects the mandible with the cranium.
- Its fibers originate in the temporal fossa and also from the deep surface of temporal fascia. Anterior fibers descend vertically whereas middle fibers run obliquely downwards and forwards and posterior fibers run horizontally forward. All these fibers converge and pass through the gap deep to the zygomatic arch and get inserted onto the medial surface, anterior border of coronoid process and anterior border of the ramus.
- *Actions* –
    d) It elevates the mandible to close the mouth
    e) It retracts the mandible after protrusion
    f) It helps in side to side grinding movement.

LATERAL PTERYGOID MUSCLE

- This masticatory muscle lies deep to the temporalis muscle and consists of upper and lower heads.
- The upper head originates from the infra temporal surface and crest of the greater wing of sphenoid bone and the lower head from the lateral surface of lateral pterygoid plate. These fibers are inserted in front of the neck of mandible and into the particular capsule and articular disc of temporomandibular joint.
- *Actions*-
    d) Depression of mandible to open the mouth.
    e) Side to side movement of the mandible.
    f) Protrusion of mandible

MEDIAL PTERYGOID MUSCLE

- It is quadrilateral and situated deep in the infra temporal fossa. It has a superficial and a deep head.
- Superficial head arises from the maxillary tuberosity and the deep head from the deep surface of lateral pterygoid plate. Fibers run downwards, backwards and laterally to get inserted into the medial surface of the angle of mandible and on the posterior part of the medial surface between the angle and the mandibular foramen.
- *Actions*-
    - d) It elevates the mandible.
    - e) It helps to protrude the mandible.
    - f) Side to side movement of the mandible.

****

Q5) Masseter.

Answer – Refer section 'Masseter' in short notes Q4 in the chapter "Mastication and Deglutition".

****

Occlusion

SHORT NOTES

Q1) Leeway space of Nance.

Answer -

- Combined mesiodistal crown width of deciduous canine, first and second molars is more than the combined mesiodistal width of their permanent successors (canine, first and second premolars). This extra space is known as Leeway space of Nance. It is present in both maxillary and mandibular arches.
- In maxilla, this space is 0.9mm on one side (total 1.8 mm in maxilla).
- In mandible, this space is 1.7mm on one side (total 3.4mm in mandible).

Importance

- This excess space helps for the mesial movements of the premolars.
- The crown of primary mandibular molars is wider mesiodistally than the crown of primary maxillary molars. Hence Leeway space is more in the mandible. Due to the space difference between the two arches, the mandibular first premolar will move more mesially than the maxillary first premolar. This movement will now change the earlier end-on relation of the deciduous molars to class I relation in the permanent dentition period.

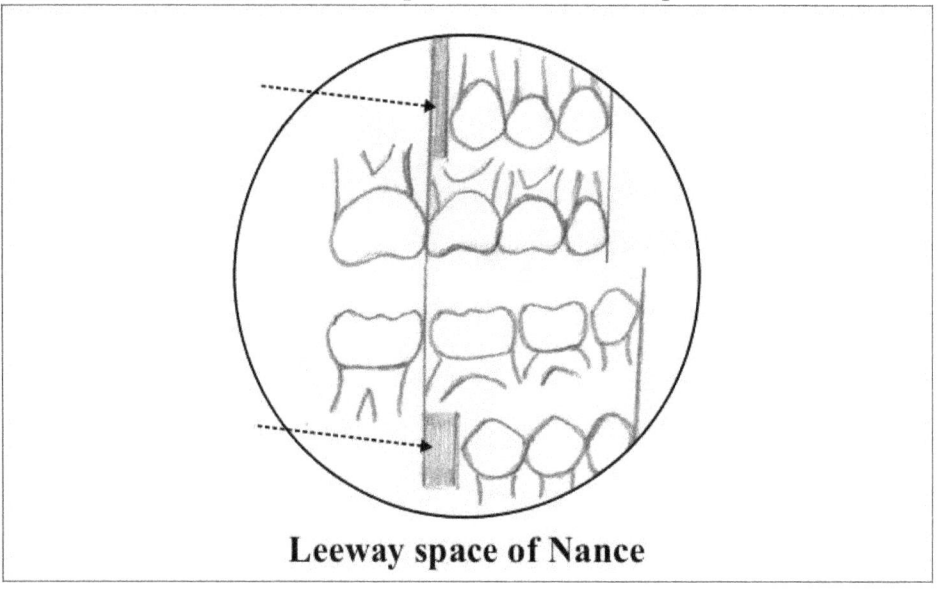

Leeway space of Nance

****

Q2) Ugly duckling stage

Answer -

- It is also called self correcting or temporary malocclusion.
- It is seen in the maxillary anterior region of children during 8-12 years of age.
- This period corresponds to the eruption of permanent maxillary canines.

- The erupting canines apply pressure on the root of lateral incisor and displace the root mesially. This in turn results in the transmission of force on the root of central incisor, which also gets mesially displaced.
- This results in the distal divergence of crowns of the two central incisors causing midline diastema. This phenomenon is known as ugly duckling stage. This is so called because children look ugly in this age group. Parents will be very concerned to get it corrected.

****

Q3) Curve of Spee.

Answer –

- Curve of Spee is a natural phenomenon seen in human dentition. The occlusal surface of upper and lower dental arches do not form a flat surface. Normally an anterioposterior curvature is required for efficient masticatory system.
- When viewed from the buccal aspect, the incisal ridges of the anterior teeth and the cusp tips of the posterior teeth form a gradual concave curve anteroposteriorly. Curve of maxillary arch is convex, and that of the mandibular arch is concave.

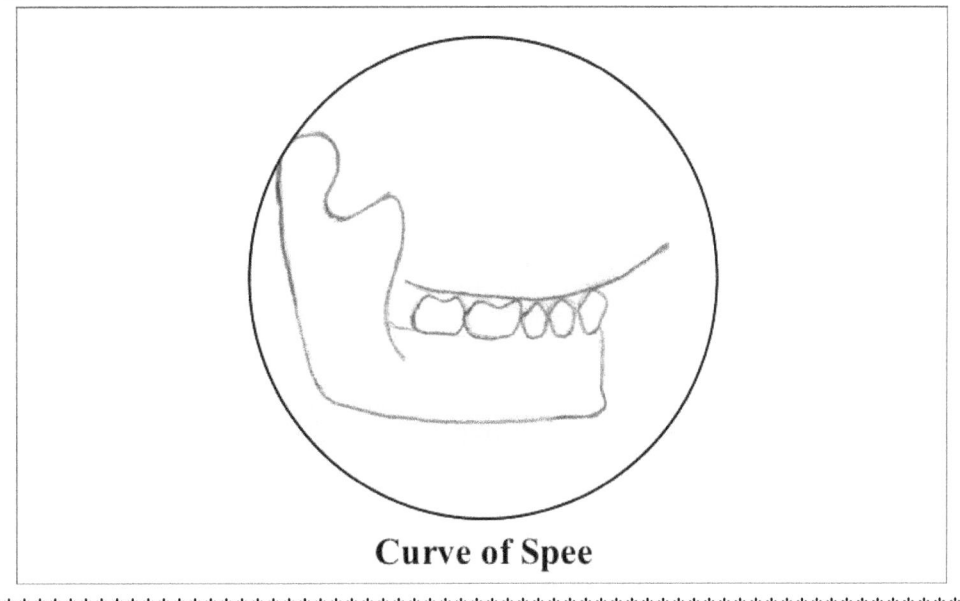

Curve of Spee

****

Q4) Curve of Wilson.

Answer – When viewed from the anterior side, the cusp tips of the posterior teeth show a smooth curvature from right to left side. This curve is known as curve of Wilson.

- The curve of maxillary arch is convex and that of mandibular arch is concave.
- The arch shows that the lingual cusps of the posterior teeth are aligned at a lower level than the buccal cusps on both sides.

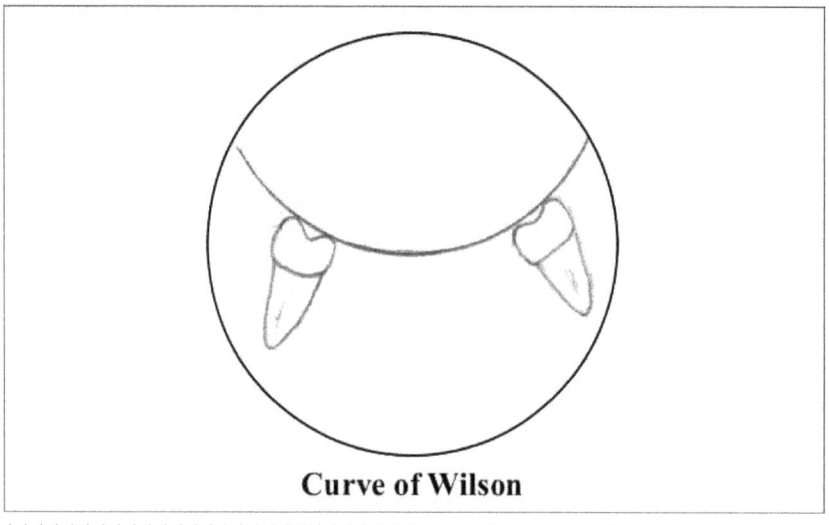

Curve of Wilson

****

Q5) Terminal plane.

Answer – A terminal plane is a line located at the end of the distal surface of the second deciduous upper and lower molars.

a) *Straight / Flush terminal plane* – mandibular deciduous second molar has a greater mesiodistal width than the maxillary deciduous second molar. Due to the difference in the dimensions of these teeth, their distal surfaces are in the same plane. This is flush terminal plane.
b) *Mesial step* – in this terminal plane relationship, the distal surface of the mandibular deciduous second molar is more mesial to the distal surface of the maxillary deciduous second molar.
c) *Distal step* – in this terminal plane relationship the distal surface of the mandibular deciduous second molar is more distal to the distal surface of the maxillary deciduous second molar.

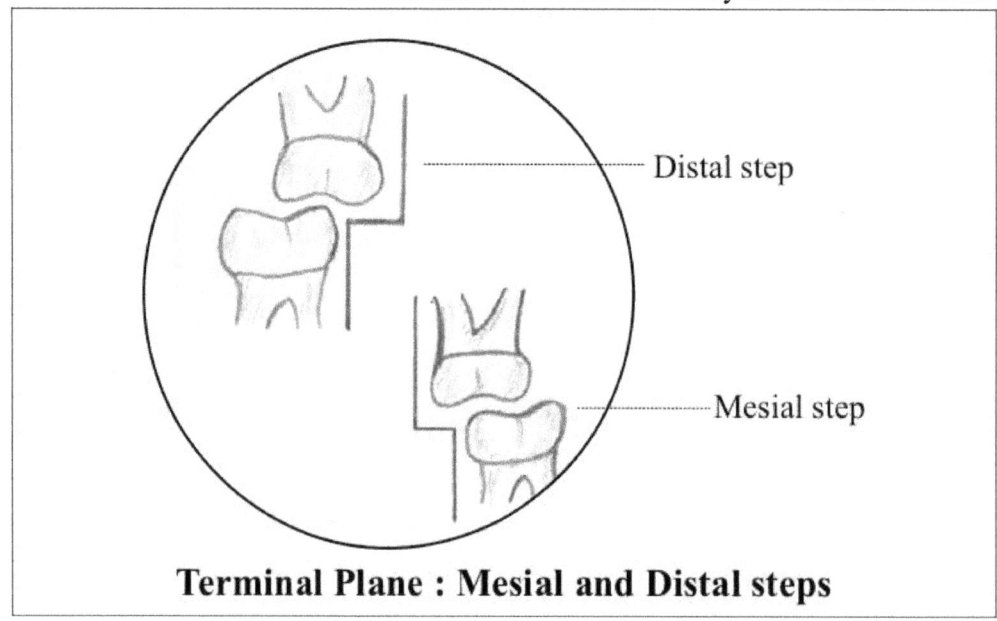

Terminal Plane : Mesial and Distal steps

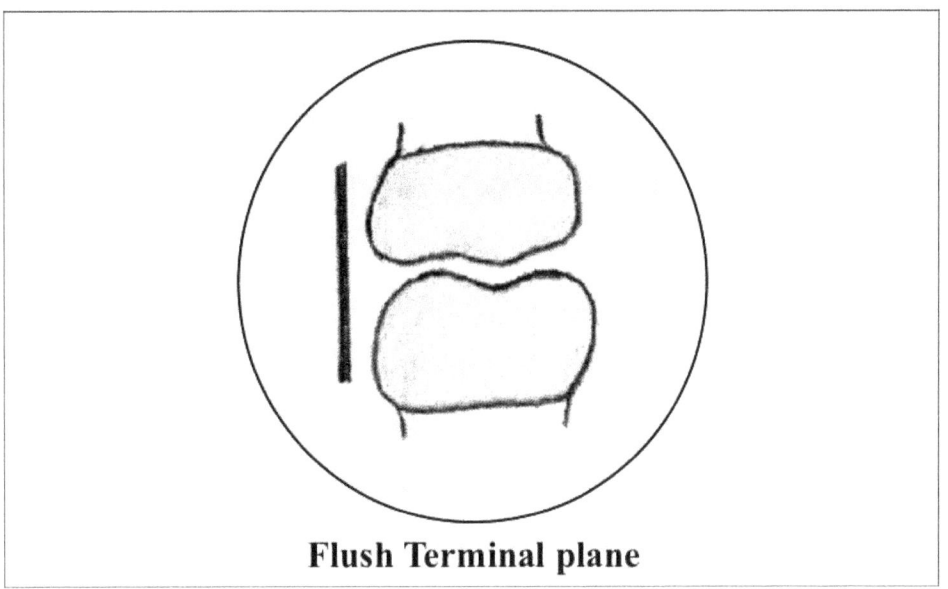

Flush Terminal plane

Importance of flush terminal plane

➢ The erupting first molars are guided by the distal surface of the deciduous second molars as they erupt into occlusion.

➢ Thus the terminal plane relationship in deciduous dentition will determine the type of molar relationship in permanent dentition.

➢ In most cases distal step leads to class II molar relationship, flush terminal plane and mesial step leads to class I molar relationship in permanent dentition.

****

Q6) Curve of Monson.

Answer –

- It is a combination of curve of Spee and the curve of Wilson in the sagittal and coronal planes.
- It is concave for mandibular and convex for maxillary teeth.
- In centric occlusion, it forms a segment of a sphere of 4 inch radius with the centre of the sphere at the glabella.

****

Oral Histology

TOOTH DEVELOPMENT

MAIN QUESTIONS

Q1) Enumerate the stages in tooth development. Discuss in detail about amelogenesis.

Answer --

MORPHOLOGICAL STAGES OF TOOTH DEVELOPMENT

- At certain points along the dental lamina, the ectodermal cells multiply at a faster rate to form knob-like structures that grow into the underlying mesenchyme. Twenty such knobs are formed that represent the tooth buds or the enamel organ of the future ten primary teeth of the maxilla and ten of the mandible. All these knobs do not appear at the same time. The first to form are those of the anterior mandible region.
- With continued cell proliferation in each enamel organ, there is an increase in size. Differential growth pattern in the enamel organ will change its shape. Tooth development will now proceed in three stages: bud, cap and bell stages.
- These terms describe only the morphology of the developing tooth germ. There is no clear distinction between these transition stages.

BUD *STAGE*

- At the site of continued localized proliferation in the dental lamina, round knob-like swellings develop, which corresponds to the position of the future deciduous teeth. This is the earliest structure of the enamel organ and is called 'tooth bud'.
- The tooth bud is lined by peripheral low cuboidal cells and central polygonal cells.
- Ectomesenchymal cells surrounding the bud undergo mitosis resulting in the condensation of these cells around the bud. This area of condensed ectomesenchyme adjacent to the bud is called *dental papilla,* from which the dentin and pulp develops. There is further condensation of ectomesenchyme surrounding both tooth bud and dental papilla is called *dental sac / follicle* which in the future form cementum.

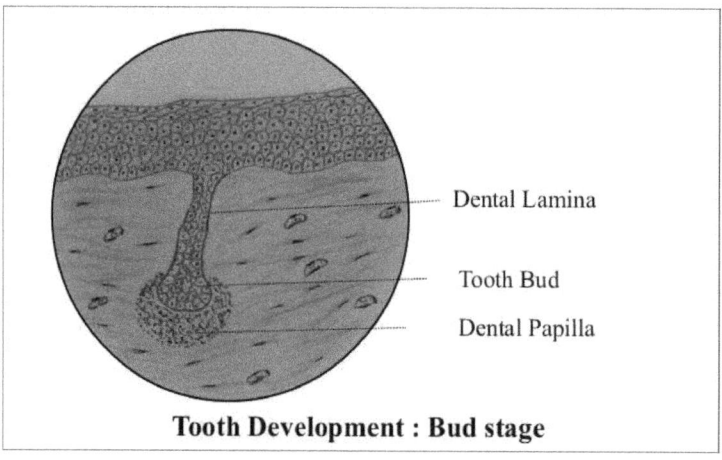

Tooth Development : Bud stage

CAP STAGE

- As the tooth bud proliferates and grows larger it does not gain a ball shape. Due to unequal growth in different parts of the tooth bud it leads to formation of cap shaped structure.
- The large epithelial growth lying over the dental papilla is now called *'enamel organ'* and it eventually forms the enamel of the tooth. The enamel organ, dental papilla and dental sac together are called the *tooth germ*.

Outer and inner enamel epithelium

- The convexity of the cap is lined by cuboidal cells and is called *outer enamel epithelium*. The inner concavity of the cap is lined by tall columnar cells and is called *inner enamel epithelium*.
- Basement membrane separates the outer enamel epithelium from the dental sac and inner enamel epithelium from the dental papilla.
- *Enamel niche* – The enamel organ appears to be attached to the overlying epithelium by double strands of dental lamina containing a core of connective tissue. It is called enamel niche. Dental lamina is a sheet rather than a single strand. A section passing through this arrangement creates the impression that the tooth germ has double attachment to the oral epithelium by two separate strands.

Stellate reticulum

- The polygonal cells located in the center of the enamel organ between the inner and outer enamel epithelium absorb water from the surrounding papilla and begin to separate. They are attached only at the point of desmosomal contact and hence appear star shaped. Now it is called stellate reticulum.
- Stellate reticulum gives cushion consistency and hence acts as a shock absorber to protect and support the delicate inner enamel epithelial cells which in future transforms into enamel forming cells (ameloblasts).
- *Enamel knot and enamel cord* -- The cells in the center of the inner enamel epithelium are densely packed to form the *enamel knot*. At the same time a vertical extension of the enamel knot develops and is called *enamel cord*. Enamel cord extends to meet the outer enamel epithelium and is termed *enamel septum*. It divides the stellate reticulum in two parts. There is a small depression at the point where the enamel septum meets outer enamel epithelium and is called *enamel naval*, (called so due to its resemblance to the umbilicus). All these structures (enamel cord, enamel septum, enamel nevus) are temporary and disappear before enamel formation. Enamel knot and enamel cord act as regulators of dividing cells for the growing enamel organ. They may also determine the shape of the tooth.

Dental papilla

- The ectomesenchyme which is enclosed in the invagination of the inner enamel epithelium undergo mitosis resulting in condensation. This area of condensed ectomesenchyme immediately

adjacent to the enamel organ is called *dental papilla* and is the formative organ of future dentin and pulp of the tooth.
- The peripheral cells of dental papilla adjacent to the inner enamel epithelium later enlarge and differentiate into dentin forming cells (odontoblasts).

Dental sac / Dental follicle

- Simultaneously with the development of the enamel organ and the dental papilla, there is condensation of the ectomesenchyme surrounding both enamel organ and the dental papilla. This is called *dental sac / follicle,* which eventually forms the supporting structures of the teeth.

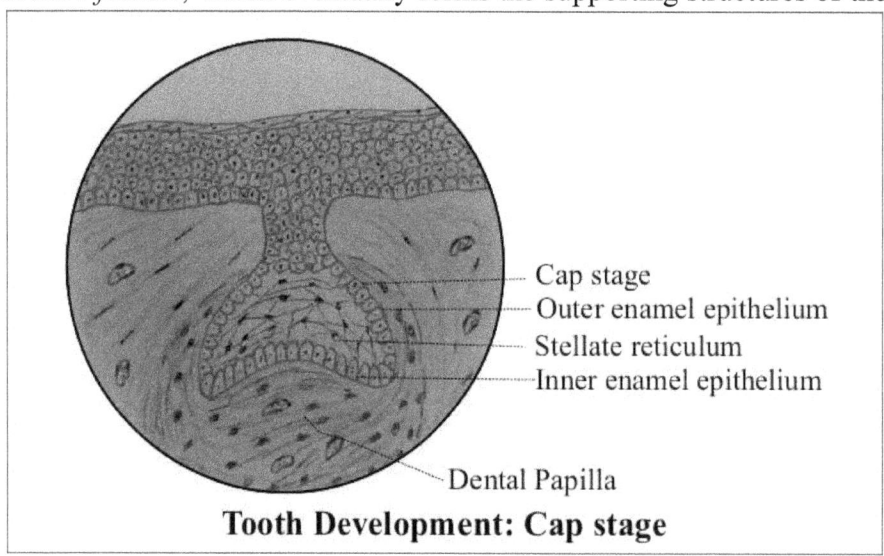

Tooth Development: Cap stage

BELL STAGE

- Continued growth of the enamel organ leads to the next stage of tooth development i.e. bell stage.
- Due to continued growth of the enamel organ there is deepening of the invagination at the margin. The enamel organ now assumes the shape of 'bell' and hence the name.
- Folding of the enamel organ to take different crown shapes could be due to the differential mitotic rate in the inner enamel epithelial cells. The shape of the crown is determined in the bell stage. In this stage the cells (ameloblasts and odontoblasts) form the hard tissues of the teeth (enamel and dentin).
- Four different types of epithelial cells can be seen enamel organ.

Inner enamel epithelium

- The inner enamel epithelium is made up of a single layer of short columnar cells that later differentiate into tall columnar ameloblasts before the beginning of amelogenesis.
- The inner enamel epithelial cells will influence the underlying dental papilla cells, which later differentiate into dentin forming cells i.e. odontoblasts.

Stratum intermedium

- Few layers of epithelial cells present between the inner enamel epithelium and stellate reticulum differentiate into a layer called stratum intermedium.
- These cells have high concentration of enzyme alkaline phosphatase (it helps for the transportation of the phosphate ions into the mineralization front).
- Stratum intermedium is not present in that part of the tooth germ that outlines the root portion of the tooth.

Stellate reticulum

- Stellate reticulum present in the center of the enamel organ expands by increase in intercellular fluid. The cells assume star-shape, with long processes that join each other.
- Before the beginning of enamel formation, the stellate reticulum collapses, to reduce the distance between the ameloblasts in the inner enamel epithelium and the source of nutrition (blood vessels) near the outer enamel epithelium.
- Now the stellate reticulum cannot be distinguished from the stratum intermedium.

Outer enamel epithelium

- The outer enamel epithelial cells of the enamel organ are now flat to low cuboidal.
- At the end of the bell stage and prior to the deposition of enamel, the outer enamel epithelium which earlier had smooth surface forms folds. Between these folds the adjacent connective tissue of the dental sac that carries rich capillary loops provides nutrition to the avascular enamel organ. This would compensate for the loss of nutritional supply from the dental papilla after the deposition of dentin.
- The zone where the outer and the inner enamel epithelium meet is known as *cervical loop*.

Dental lamina

- Lingual extension of dental lamina is seen in the early bell stage and is termed *successional lamina* as it gives rise to the enamel organs of the successor (permanent) teeth.
- Enamel organs of the deciduous teeth will be in the bell stage and their successor teeth in the bud stage.

Dental papilla

- The dental papilla is enclosed in the invaginated portion of the enamel organ.
- Before the inner enamel epithelial cells differentiate into ameloblasts and lay down enamel, the peripheral cells of the dental papilla adjacent to the inner enamel epithelium differentiate into odontoblasts under the influence of inner enamel epithelial cells.
- Initially these cells will be cuboidal, but later assume columnar shape with changes in their functional activity.
- Once the dentin formation begins, the dental papilla will be designated as dental pulp.

Dental sac

- The dental sac encloses the enamel organ and the dental papilla.
- With the development of the root the fibers in the dental sac differentiate into periodontal ligament fibers. They become embedded in the developing cementum and bone.

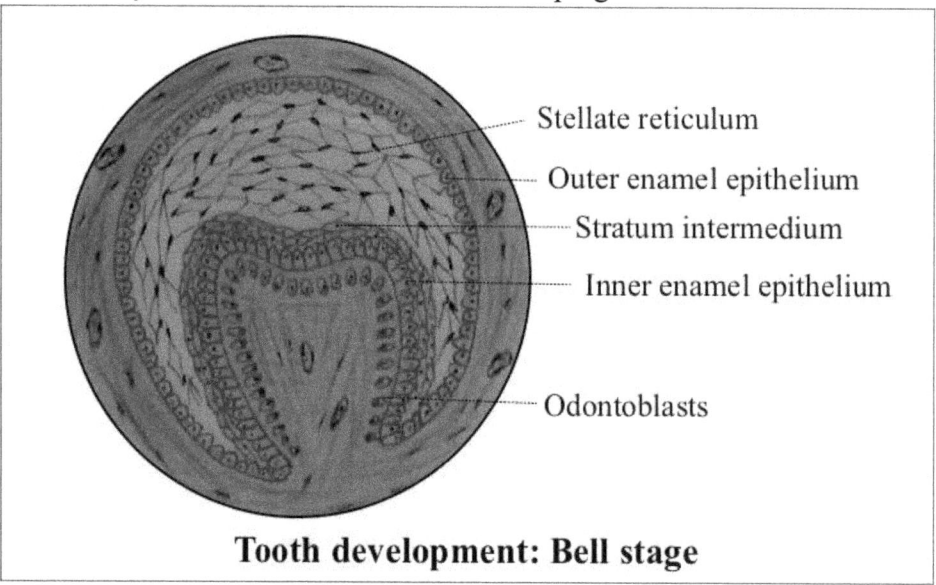

Tooth development: Bell stage

ADVANCED BELL STAGE

- This stage is characterized by the beginning of mineralization and root formation.
- The boundary between inner enamel epithelium and odontoblasts will be the future dentinoenamel junction (DEJ).
- Deposition of dentin first begins on the DEJ in the region of future incisal edge or the cusp tip. From here the deposition proceeds pulpally and apically.
- Once first layer of dentin is deposited, the inner enamel epithelial cells differentiate into ameloblasts and lay down enamel over the dentin. The deposition of enamel begins from the incisal edge or the cusp tip. The enamel deposition now proceeds upwards from the DEJ towards the surface.
- The cervical portion of the enamel organ gives rise to Hertwig's epithelial root sheath from which the root develops. This root sheath consists of two layers of cells (inner and outer enamel epithelial cells). It is responsible for the shape, length and number of roots.
- Dental lamina connecting the tooth germ to the oral epithelium fragments thus separating the developing tooth from the oral epithelium. Normally these epithelial fragments degenerate. But some may persist as remnants (cell rests of Serrae).

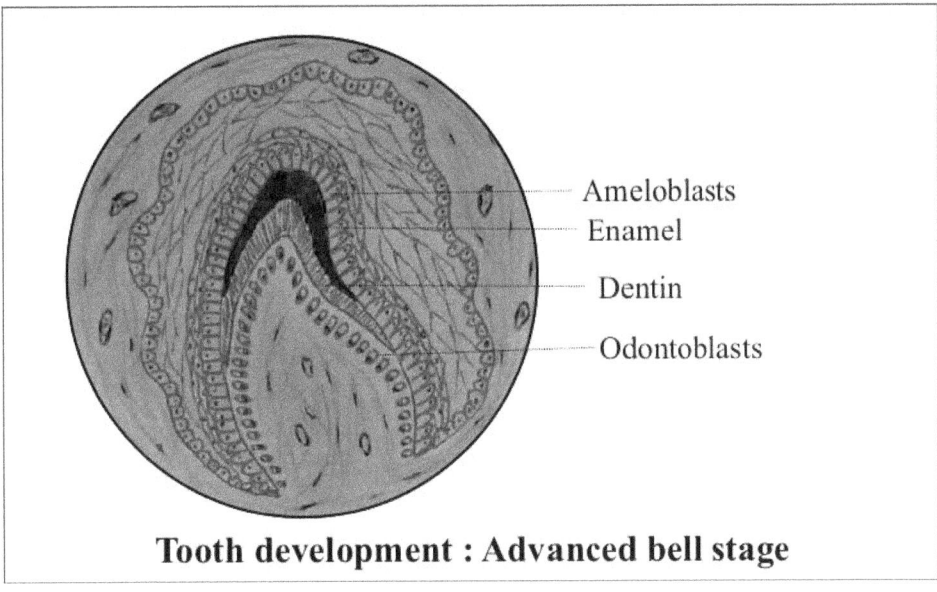

Tooth development : Advanced bell stage

PHYSIOLOGICAL STAGES OF TOOTH DEVELOPMENT

- Various physiological processes take place during tooth development. These processes overlap and are continuous throughout the morphological stages.

Initiation

- Dental lamina has specific cells that have the potential to form enamel organ under the influence of certain factors that initiate or induce tooth development. Different teeth are initiated at different times.
- Such an initiation to form an enamel organ requires epithelial-mesenchymal interactions. Although mechanism for such interactions is not clearly understood, experimentally it has been proved that mesenchyme of the dental papilla can instruct the tooth epithelium or even nontooth epithelium to form tooth.

Proliferation

- Once tooth formation is initiated, there is increased proliferative activity ultimately resulting in the bud, cap and bell stages of the enamel organ.
- Proliferative growth leads to increase in size and proportion of the tooth germ.

Histodifferentiation

- Proliferative stage is succeeded by the histodifferentiation stage.
- This phase is very active during bell stage, just before the beginning of formation and apposition of dentin and enamel.
- The formative cells of the tooth germ (inner enamel epithelial cells and dental papilla) undergo specific morphologic and functional changes. As they differentiate, they give up their capacity to divide and assume their new function to produce either dentin or enamel matrix.

- Organizing influence of the inner enamel epithelial cells on the adjacent mesenchymal cells of the dental papilla results in its differentiation into odontoblasts.
- As the odontoblasts begin secreting dentin, the inner enamel epithelial cells differentiate into ameloblasts and lay enamel matrix over the preformed dentin.
- Experiments have proved that enamel is not formed in the absence of dentin. Hence dentin is essential for enamel formation.
- Differentiation of the odontoblasts is essential for initiation of dentin formation and later differentiation of ameloblasts and enamel formation.

Morphodifferentiation

- In the morphodifferentiation stage, differential growth within the tooth germ decides the size and morphologic pattern of the future tooth.
- In the advanced bell stage there is both active histodifferentiation and morphodifferentiation taking place.
- The size and form of the cusp is established much before the deposition of the dental hard tissues.

Apposition

- Apposition means deposition of the matrix of the dental hard tissues.
- In the apposition stage, deposition of the hard tissues of the tooth i.e. enamel, dentin and cementum takes place.
- Appositional growth is characterized by regular, rhythmic deposition of extracellular matrix of enamel, dentin and cementum. Periods of activity and rest alternate at definite intervals at the time of deposition.

For 'Amelogenesis' refer main question Q2 in chapter "Enamel".

****

Q2) Enumerate the stages in tooth development and write on advanced bell stage of tooth development with suitable diagrams.

Answer – Refer main question Q1 in chapter "Tooth development".

****

Q3) Write in detail the histology of tooth germ during the stages of tooth development.

Answer –

BUD STAGE

- The tooth bud consists of peripheral low cuboidal cells and central polygonal cells.
- The ectomesenchymal cells underlying the tooth bud shows condensation. This area of condensed ectomesenchyme immediately adjacent to the tooth bud is called *dental papilla*. The

condensed ectomsenchyme surrounding both tooth bud and dental papilla is called *dental sac/follicle*.

CAP STAGE

Epithelium

- The convexity of the cap is lined by cuboidal cells and is called *outer enamel epithelium*. The inner concavity of the cap is lined by tall columnar cells and is called *inner enamel epithelium.*
- Basement membrane separates the outer enamel epithelium from the dental sac and inner enamel epithelium from the dental papilla.
- *Enamel niche* – The enamel organ appears to be attached to the overlying epithelium by double strands of dental lamina having a containing a core of connective tissue. It is called enamel niche. Dental lamina is a sheet rather than a single strand. A section passing through this arrangement creates the impression that the tooth germ has double attachment to the oral epithelium by two separate strands.

Stellate reticulum

- The polygonal cells located in the center of the enamel organ between the inner and outer enamel epithelium absorb water from the surrounding papilla and begin to separate. They are attached only at the point of desmosomal contact and hence appear star shaped. Now it is called stellate reticulum.
- *Enamel knot and enamel cord* -- The cells in the center of the inner enamel epithelium are densely packed to form the *enamel knot*. At the same time a vertical extension of the enamel knot occurs and is called *enamel cord*. Enamel cord extends to meet the outer enamel epithelium and is termed *enamel septum*. It divides the stellate reticulum in two parts. There is a small depression at the point where the enamel septum meets outer enamel epithelium and is called *enamel naval*, (called so due to its resemblance to the umbilicus). All these structures are temporary and disappear before enamel formation starts.

Dental papilla

- The ectomesenchyme which is enclosed in the invagination of the inner enamel epithelium undergo mitosis resulting in condensation. This area of condensed ectomesenchyme immediately adjacent to the enamel organ is called *dental papilla*. Budding capillaries and mitotic figures are seen the dental papilla.

Dental sac / Dental follicle

- Marginal condensation of the ectomesenchyme surrounding both enamel organ and the dental papilla is called *dental sac / follicle*.

EARLY BELL STAGE

- The enamel organ assumes the shape of 'bell' and hence the name. Four different types of epithelial cells can be seen enamel organ.

  a) *Inner enamel epithelium* -- The inner enamel epithelium is a single layer of short columnar / cuboidal cells.

  b) *Stratum intermedium* -- These are a few layers of squamous cells between the inner enamel epithelium and the stellate reticulum. This layer is not present in the part of the tooth germ that outlines the root portion of the tooth.

  c) *Stellate reticulum* -- These cells are star-shape, with long processes that join with each other. Before the beginning of enamel formation, the stellate reticulum collapses, to reduce the distance between the ameloblasts in the inner enamel epithelium and the outer enamel epithelium. Now it cannot be distinguished from the stratum intermedium.

  d) *Outer enamel epithelium* -- The outer enamel epithelial cells are flat to low cuboidal. At the end of the bell stage and prior to the deposition of enamel, the outer enamel epithelium which earlier had smooth surface forms folds. Between these folds the adjacent connective tissue of the dental sac will have rich capillary loops. The zone where the outer and the inner enamel epithelium meet is known as *cervical loop.*

- *Dental papilla* – the peripheral cells of dental papilla are tall columnar (odontoblasts).
- *Dental sac* -- The dental sac encloses the enamel organ and the dental papilla. Fibers in the dental sac differentiate into periodontal ligament fibers. They become embedded in the developing cementum and bone.
- *Dental lamina*-- Lingual extension of dental lamina is seen in the early bell stage and is termed *successional lamina* as it gives rise to the enamel organs of the successor (permanent) teeth. Enamel organs of the deciduous teeth will be in the bell stage and their successor teeth in the bud stage.

ADVANCED BELL STAGE

- This stage is characterized by the beginning of mineralization and root formation.
- The boundary between inner enamel epithelium and odontoblasts will be the future dentinoenamel junction (DEJ).
- Deposition of dentin first begins on the DEJ in the region of future incisal edge or the cusp tip. From here the deposition proceeds pulpally and apically.
- Once first layer of dentin is deposited, the inner enamel epithelial cells differentiate into ameloblasts and lay down enamel over the dentin. The deposition of enamel begins from the incisal edge or the cusp tip. The enamel deposition now proceeds upwards from the DEJ towards the surface.
- The cervical portion of the enamel organ gives rise to Hertwig's epithelial root sheath from which the root develops. This root sheath consists of two layers of cells (inner and outer enamel epithelial cells). It is responsible for the shape, length and number of roots.

- Dental lamina connecting the tooth germ to the oral epithelium fragments thus separating the developing tooth from the oral epithelium. Normally these epithelial fragments degenerate. But some may persist as remnants (cell rests of Serrae).

****

SHORT NOTES

Q1) Dental lamina and its fate.

Q) Primary epithelial band and dental lamina.

Answer -- The primitive oral cavity is lined by stratified epithelium called oral ectoderm. This oral ectoderm contacts the endoderm of the foregut to form the buccopharyngeal membrane. At about twenty-seventh day, this membrane ruptures and primitive oral cavity gets connected with the foregut.

- Two to three weeks after the rupture of the buccopharyngeal membrane, basal cells in certain areas of the oral ectoderm proliferate rapidly than the cells in the adjacent area leading to the formation of primary epithelial band. This band of thickened epithelium is continuous, horseshoe-shaped and is formed in the site of future upper and lower jaws.
- Later the primary epithelial band divides into inner extension called dental lamina and outer extension called vestibular lamina. Dental lamina forms slightly before the vestibular lamina.
- Successors of primary teeth (i.e., permanent anteriors and premolars) develop from the lingual extension of the dental lamina, opposite to the developing enamel organ of the deciduous tooth. This lingual extension of the dental lamina is called successional lamina. Later with the growth of the jaws, distal proliferation of the dental lamina occurs from which the tooth buds of permanent molars develop.

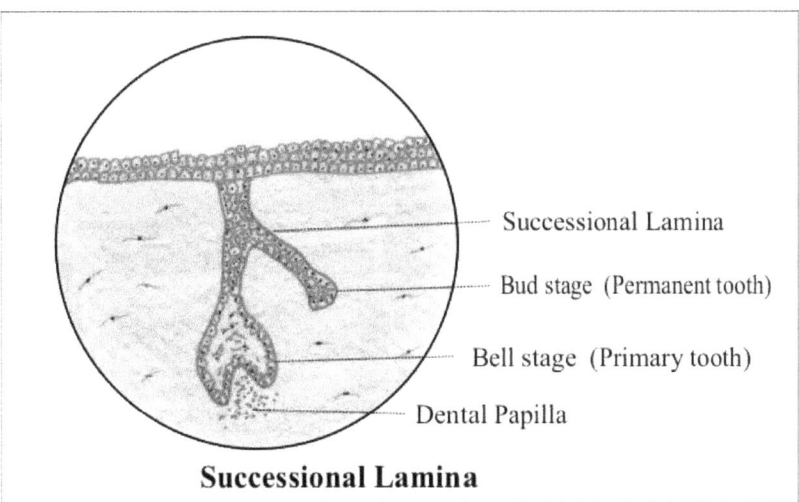

Successional Lamina

Fate of dental lamina

- Activity of dental lamina persists for a period of five years.

- After the initiation of tooth development, dental lamina connecting the tooth germ to the oral epithelium fragments thus separating the developing tooth from the oral epithelium. Normally these epithelial fragments degenerate. But some may persist as remnants within the jaws and gingiva as epithelial pearls or islands and are called *cell rests of Serres*.

****

Q2) Hertwig's epithelial root sheath (HERS).

Answer –

- Development of the root begins after enamel and dentin formation has reached the future cementoenamel junction.
- The zone in the tooth germ where the outer and the inner enamel epithelium meet is known as *cervical loop*. Once the crown formation is complete, the inner and the outer enamel epithelial cells at the cervical loop of the enamel organ proliferate to form a double layer strand called Hertwig's epithelial root sheath (HERS). HERS plays an important role in determining the shape of the root and initiating root dentin formation.
- HERS extends between the dental papilla and the dental follicle. The cells of the inner layer of HERS are cuboidal and do not produce enamel. They initiate the differentiation of the adjacent ectomesenchymal cells of the dental papilla into odontoblasts, which forms the root dentin.
- With the deposition of root dentin, the connective tissue of the dental follicle that surrounds the root sheath proliferates and invades the root sheath. Root sheath loses its continuity and degenerates. Some persist as remnants in the periodontal ligament as epithelial islands or strands and are called as *'cell rests of Malassez'*. The dental follicle cells differentiate into cementoblasts and lay down cementum over the newly formed dentin.

****

Q3) Physiologic stages of tooth development.

Answer – Refer section 'Physiologic stages of tooth development' in main question Q1 in chapter "Tooth development".

****

Q5) Enamel knot and enamel cord

Q) Transient structures of enamel organ.

Answer -- In the cap stage of tooth development, the enamel organ appears like a cap. It has three layers – inner enamel epithelium, outer enamel epithelium and stellate reticulum in-between. The cells in the center of the inner enamel epithelium are densely packed to form the *enamel knot*. At the same time a vertical extension of the enamel knot called *enamel cord* also occurs. Enamel cord extends to meet the outer enamel epithelium and is termed *enamel septum,* as it divides the stellate reticulum in two parts. There is a small depression at the point where the enamel septum meets outer enamel epithelium and is called *enamel naval,* due to its resemblance to the umbilicus. All these structures are temporary and disappear before enamel formation starts. Enamel knot and enamel cord may act as reservoir of dividing cells for the growing enamel organ. They may also determine the shape of the tooth.

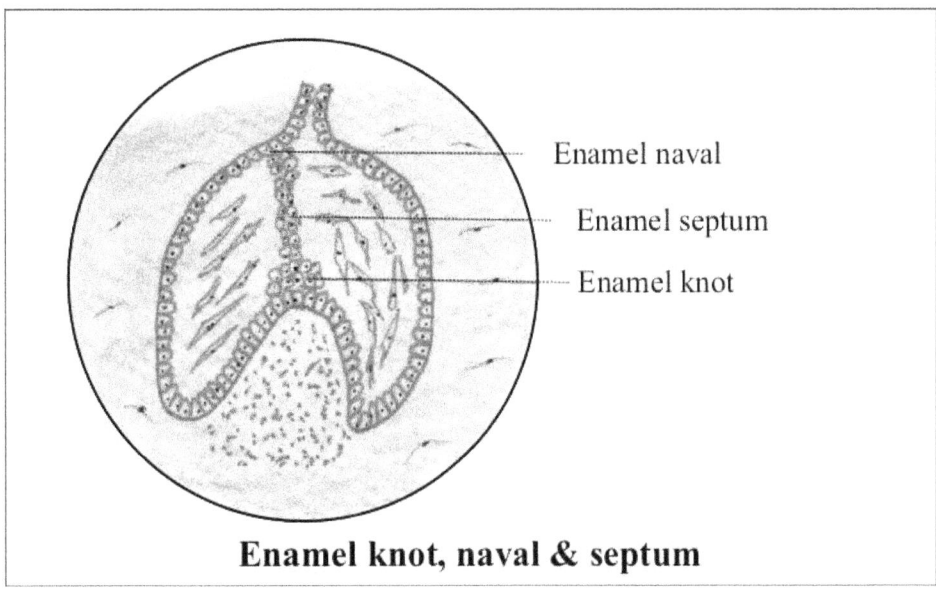

Enamel knot, naval & septum

ENAMEL

MAIN QUESTIONS

Q1) Describe the stages in the life cycle of ameloblasts with suitable diagrams.

Answer–Ameloblasts are the cells responsible for enamel development and maturation.

The life span of ameloblasts can be divided into six stages

- a) Morphogenic stage
- b) Organizing stage
- c) Formative stage
- d) Maturative stage
- e) Protective stage
- f) Desmolytic stage

MORPHOGENIC STAGE

- Before ameloblasts differentiate from the inner enamel epithelial cells (IEE) and begin enamel synthesis, they first communicate with the adjacent mesenchymal cells of the dental papilla to determine the crown's morphology.
- The inner enamel epithelial cells exhibit a short or low columnar morphology during the morphogenic phase, with big oval nuclei that almost completely fill the cell body.

ORGANIZING STAGE

- During the organizing phase, the IEE cells (future ameloblasts) undergo morphological alterations. They become tall columnar. There is migration of golgi bodies and centrioles from the proximal end (i.e., the cell end facing stratum intermedium) of the cell into the distal end (i.e. the cell end facing dentin).
- Before ameloblasts differentiate from the IEE cells and begin enamel formation, they first interact with adjacent mesenchymal cells of the dental papilla to define the crown's morphology.
- Consequently, the elimination of the cell-free zone brought about by elongation of cells facilitates contact between the inner enamel epithelial cells and the dental papilla cells. The epithelial-mesenchymal interaction begins, resulting in the development of odontoblasts from the cells of dental papilla.
- At the termination of the organizing stage, odontoblasts begin the secretion of dentin. The initial appearance of dentin is a crucial stage in the developmental cycle of the IEE cells. They then develop into ameloblasts.

- Provided that the inner enamel epithelial cells maintain contact with the connective tissue (CT) of dental papilla, the blood vessels present there provide nutrient materials to it. When dentin forms, the nutrient supply is cut off. The outer enamel epithelium (OEE) is thrown into folds. The distance between the capillaries in the CT that surrounds the OEE and the stratum intermedium and the ameloblasts is shortened. Nutrients are now obtained from these capillaries.

FORMATIVE STAGE

- Upon the formation of the dentin's initial layer, the transformation of inner enamel epithelial cells into ameloblasts begin.
- Dentin is important for the initiation of enamel matrix development.
- The ameloblasts maintain consistent length and shape during enamel matrix production. Ameloblasts form blunt cellular processes that penetrate the basal lamina (BL) and extend into the predentin.
- Before ameloblasts differentiate from the IEE cells and begin enamel formation, they first communicate with neighboring mesenchymal cells of the dental papilla to define the crown's morphology.

MATURATIVE STAGE

- Enamel maturation (complete mineralization) commences following the formation of the majority of enamel matrix thickness in occlusal or incisal region.
- The creation of the enamel matrix is still occurring in the cervical region of the crown at this stage.
- At the termination of this stage, the height of the ameloblasts is marginally diminished and they are closely adhered to the enamel matrix.
- Stratum intermedium (SI) cells undergo a transformation from a cuboidal morphology to a spindle shape.

PROTECTIVE STAGE

- Upon complete deposition and calcification of the enamel, the ameloblasts are organized into a distinct layer. It is indistinguishable from the cells of the SI and OEE.
- The outer enamel epithelium, stratum intermedium, along with ameloblast subsequently creates a stratified epithelial layer over the enamel, referred to as *reduced enamel epithelium (REE)*.
- *Function of reduced enamel epithelium*-- Until the tooth emerges, the developed enamel is protected by being isolated from the connective tissue. Anomalies could appear if the connective tissue and enamel come into contact. [i.e., enamel may be resorbed or cementum may be deposited].

DESMOLYTIC STAGE

- During the desmolyticstage, the REE undergoes proliferation and merges with the oral epithelium. The cells at the core of this fused epithelium undergo degeneration due to insufficient nutrition, resulting in a perforation that facilitates tooth eruption.
- The premature degradation of REE may inhibit tooth eruption.

****

Q2) Describe amelogenesis in detail.

Answer – The mechanism of enamel formation is termed amelogenesis.

- Amelogenesis is a lengthy process that may require up to 5 years to finalize in certain teeth.
- Before ameloblasts differentiate from the IEE cells and begin enamel formation, they first communicate with the adjacent mesenchymal cells of the dental papilla to define the crown's morphology.
- In the life cycle of ameloblasts, enamel formation happens during the formative and maturative stages and coincides with the late bell stage of tooth development.

Amelogenesis is subdivided into three main functional stages

    a) Presecretory stage.

    b) Secretory stage.

    c) Mineralization andMaturative stage.

Stage 1: Presecretory stage

▶ During the presecretory phase, several changes in morphology are apparent inside the cells of the IEE before they transform into ameloblasts.

▶ Before ameloblasts start enamel formation, they first communicate with adjacent mesenchymal cells of the dental papilla to define the crown's morphology.

▶ Upon the deposition of dentin, the IEE cells undergo differentiation into ameloblasts. They develop into tall columnar cells and their nuclei migrate proximally (i.e., towards the SI). The Golgi complex and rough endoplasmic reticulum (rER) expand in volume and migrate towards the distal end (i.e., towards the dentin).

▶ Changes in the ameloblasts indicate their synthetic and secretory functions.

▶ The IEE cell differentiation initiates at cusp tip or incisal edge and there after progresses down the slopes of tooth crown until all cells have transformed into ameloblasts.

Stage 2: Secretory stage

▶ Ribosomes in ameloblasts produce enamel proteins. The proteins are subsequently transported to the golgi complex, where they are modified and contained into secretory granules.

▶ The granules translocate to the distal aspect of the cell (i.e., toward dentin), and their contents are discharged against the freshly created mantle dentin to create a thin layer of enamel.

▶ Enamel development begins at the cusp tip or incisal edge and there after descends along the cusp slope. The IEE cells at the cusp tip or incisal edge were the initial cells to develop into ameloblasts.

▶ The mineralization of the newly produced enamel matrix begins immediately. The first generated hydroxyapatite crystals in the enamel interdigitate with those in the dentin.

▶ Upon the formation of the enamel layer, ameloblasts migrate upwards from the dentin surface.

▶ Ameloblasts now experience significant morphological alterations to prepare for their subsequent functional role, namely, the mineralization and maturation of enamel. They diminish in length, accompanied by a reduction in volume and organelle content.

Stage 3: Mineralization and Maturation stage

▶ The maturation phase is significantly longer than the secretory phase.

▶ In the maturing phase, the height of ameloblasts diminishes, and enamel secretion ceases entirely. The primary function of ameloblasts is to eliminate water and organic compounds from enamel matrix while incorporating inorganic materials.

- During the maturation stage, ameloblasts exhibit ruffled and smooth-ended boundaries in contact with the enamel surface.
- The ruffled-ended ameloblasts facilitate calcium influx into the developing enamel, whereas the smooth-ended ameloblasts enable the expulsion of proteins and water from the enamel matrix.
- Upon deposition, enamel experiences rapid mineralization of up to 30%. Upon the complete formation of enamel thickness, an increased deposition of minerals occurs along side the elimination of enamel proteins and water, culminating in a more mineralized layer.
- Maturation at the ultrastructural level is seen as the crystals growth due to incorporation of minerals.
- Following the maturation phase, approximately 50% of ameloblasts experience apoptosis. Autophagocytosis occurs in organelles involved in protein production.
- Ameloblasts deposit basal lamina (referred to as enamel cuticle or Nasmyth's membrane) over the newly created enamel surface and adhere to it through hemidesmosomes.

****

Q3) Describe in detail the hypocalcified structures in enamel.

Answer – The hypocalcified structures inside enamel are……

a) **_Rod sheath_**–Enamel rods constitute the fundamental structural components of enamel. In an electron microscope, rods or prisms are protected by a rod sheath and defined by interrod material. When sectioned longitudinally, the cuts traverse the "heads" or "bodies" of one row of rods and the "tails" of an adjacent row. This creates an appearance of rods being divided by interrod material. The "bodies" of the rods are oriented towards the occlusal or incisal surface, while the "tails" are directed cervically.

b)   Incremental lines of Retzius (refer to short notes Q5, in chapter "Enamel").

c)   Enamel lamellae (refer short notes Q3, in chapter "Enamel").

d)   Enamel tufts (refer short notes Q2, in chapter "Enamel").

e)   Neonatal line (refer short notes Q6, in chapter "Enamel").

f)   Enamel spindles (refer short notes Q10, in chapter "Enamel").

g)   Enamel cracks (refer short notes Q18, in chapter "Enamel").

****

SHORT NOTES

Q1) Enamel rods / Enamel prisms.

Answer -- Enamel rods/prisms are the basic structural units forming the enamel.

Number – Number of enamel rods varies from tooth to tooth.

Direction -- The rods are positioned perpendicularly to dentin surface.

- In both cervical region and the central portions of a deciduous tooth's crown, they are oriented horizontally.
- In the cervical region of the permanent tooth, the rods deviate in the apical direction. Whereas in the central part of the crown, they are horizontal.
- They are oriented vertically in the area of the incisal edge or cusp tip.
- On the cusp tip or the incisal edge, bundles of rods appear to interlace with each other in an irregular fashion. The optical phenomenon of enamel is referred to as *gnarled enamel*.

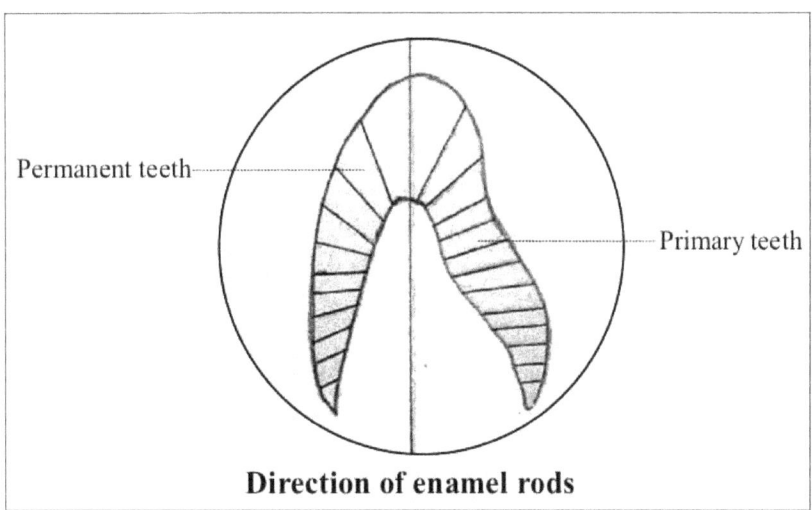

Direction of enamel rods

Course – The rod follows a wavy course. The rod's length exceeds the enamel's thickness. The rods at the cusp tip/incisal edge are longer than those in the cervical area.

Diameter -- The rod's diameter expands from dentinoenamel junction (DEJ) to the enamel surface.

Appearance -- The enamel rods exhibit a distinct crystalline appearance, allowing light to permeate through them. In cross-sections of human teeth, enamel prisms exhibit a resemblance to fish scales.

Ultrastructure -- In an electron microscope, rods or prisms are enclosed by a rod sheath and separated by inter-rod material.

- A common configuration is a keyhole or paddle-shaped prism within human enamel. The patterns differ throughout various regions of the enamel.

- When sectioned longitudinally, the cuts traverse the 'heads' or 'bodies' of one row of rods and the 'tails' of a neighboring row. This creates the appearance of interrod material filled between rods heads.
- The 'bodies' of the rods are oriented towards the occlusal or incisal surface, while their tail's are directed cervically.
- The hydroxyapatite crystals within the rods are oriented nearly parallel to the rods' long axis, deviating around 65 degrees as they extend into the prism's tail.

Striations --Every enamel rod is composed of segments defined by dark lines, resulting in a "striated" appearance. The rods are segmented due to the rhythmic development of the enamel matrix. These segments are uniform in length.

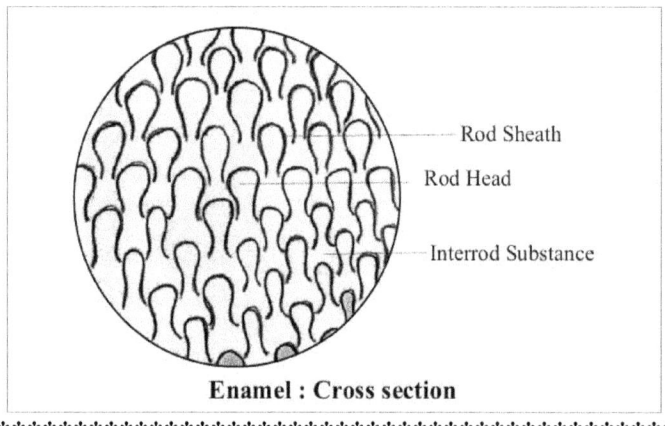

Enamel : Cross section

****

Q2) Enamel tufts.

Answer --Enamel tufts are hypomineralized enamel prisms with interprismatic material. They are elongated, ribbon-like structures that begin at the DEJ and extend into the enamel for a significant distance. They are named thus due to their similarity to tufts of grass. They extend along the long axis of the crown, thereby exhibiting better view in horizontal or cross-section of tooth. They have a higher concentration of enamel proteins relative to the rest of the enamel.

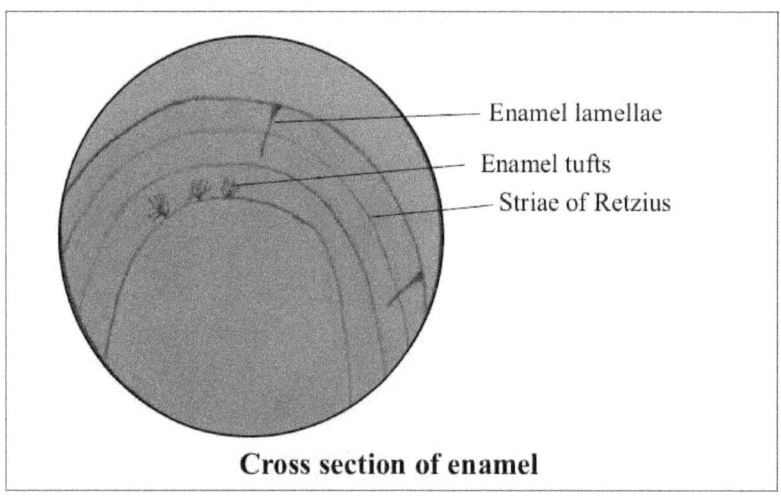

Cross section of enamel

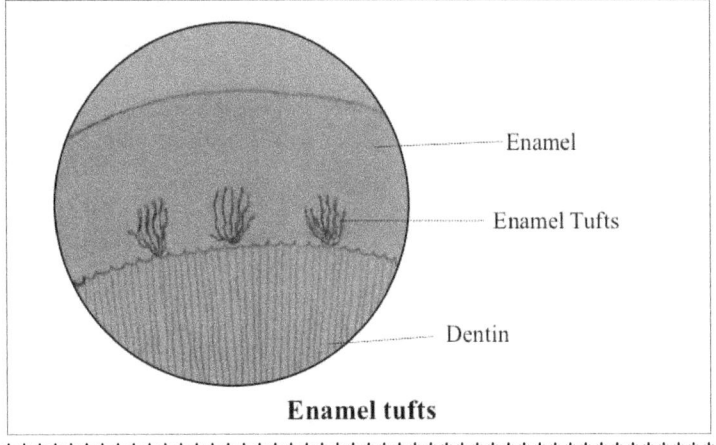
Enamel tufts

****

Q3) Enamel lamellae.

Answer–Enamel lamellae are elongated, leaf-like, hypomineralized structures that extend from the enamel surface to the DEJ and at times into the dentin.

- They comprise of organic matter with few inorganic constituents.
- Lamellae extend along the long axis of the crown, making them better visible in horizontal or cross-sectional view of the teeth.

There are 3 types of lamellae

a) Type A: lamellae consisting of inadequately calcified rod segments.
b) Type B: lamellae composed of degenerated cells.
c) Type C: lamellae arising in erupted teeth.

- Type A may be confined to enamel, while types B and C can extend into the dentin.
- *Significance* -- Enamel lamellae may signify a site of susceptibility in a tooth. It acts as a route for bacterial entry into the tooth, potentially leading to caries.

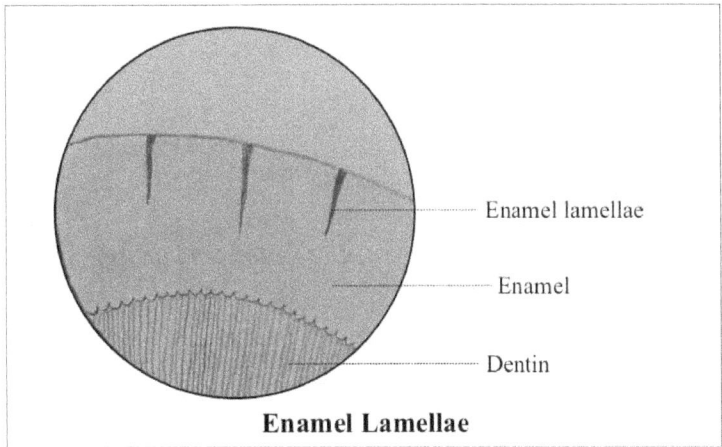
Enamel Lamellae

****

Q4) Hunter Schreger bands.

▶ **Answer** –Bands of Hunter Schreger are apparent phenomena distinguished by alternating dark and light zones found in the inner two-thirds of enamel. They are best observed in a longitudinal section of the tooth under oblique reflected light.

▶ The consistent alteration in enamel rods orientation is considered a functional adaptation to mitigate the danger of fracture from masticatory stresses. The alteration in the orientation of enamel rods accounts for the appearance of Hunter-Schreger bands.

▶ The dark bands are classified as *diazones*. The light bands are referred to as *parazones*.

▶ These bands start at the dentinoenamel junction and continue outward and upward to a specific distance within the enamel.

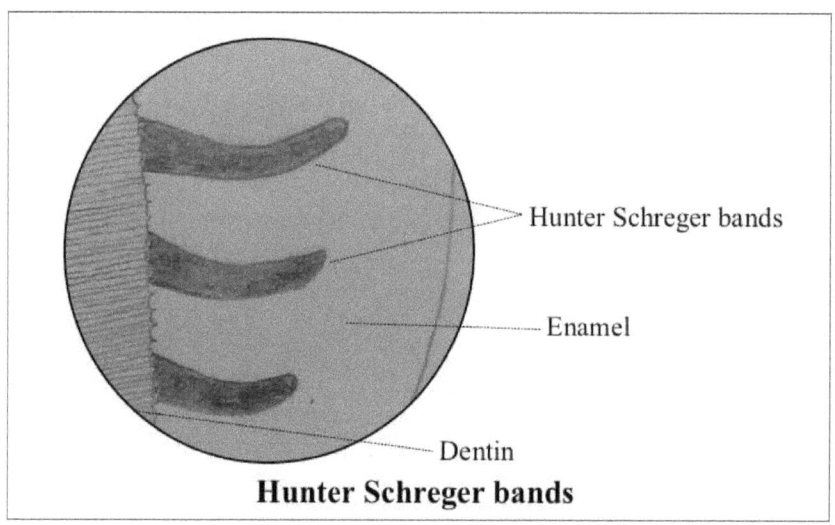

Hunter Schreger bands

****

Q5) Incremental lines of Retzius.

Answer –The striae of Retzius signify the progressive deposition of enamel matrix during amelogenesis.

▶ It appears as brownish streaks.
▶ They start at the dentinoenamel junction and as they traverse the enamel, they diverge occlusally.
▶ In longitudinal section, they are observed around the apex of pulp horn at the incisal edge or on cusp tip.
▶ In the cervical region, they traverse more obliquely.
▶ In a transverse section of the tooth, it appears as concentric circles, akin to the annular rings observed in the cross-section of a tree.
▶ Incremental lines indicate differences in structure and mineralization, either hypo- or hyper-mineralization, during enamel creation.

▸ The neonatal line is distinct striae of Retzius. The darkening of the striae seems to occur from abrupt changes in the newborn neonate's environment and nutrition. Neonatal lines are also generated by metabolic abnormalities that impact amelogenesis.

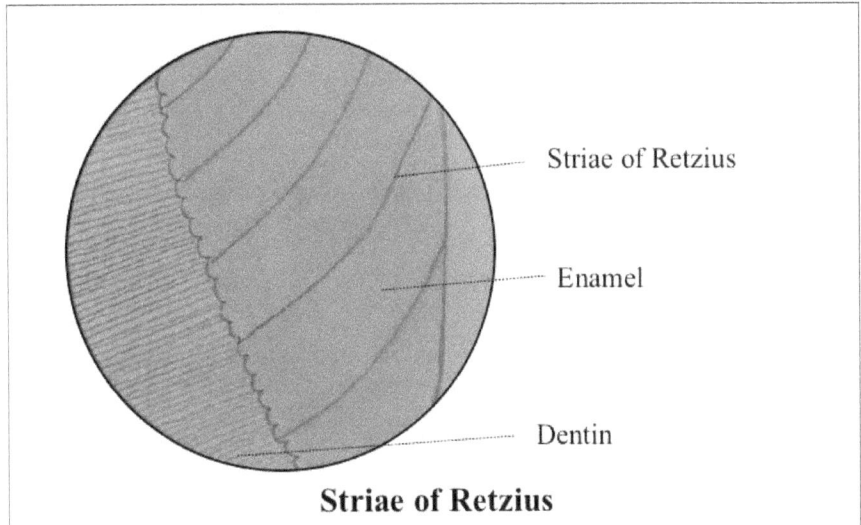

Striae of Retzius

****

Q6) Neonatal line.

▸ **Answer** --The enamel of deciduous teeth forms partially before birth (prenatal enamel) and partially after birth (postnatal enamel). The boundary between pre- and postnatal enamel in deciduous teeth is indicated by a prominent incremental line of Retzius referred to as the neonatal line or ring.

▸ The darkening of the striae of Retzius seems to occur from abrupt changes in the environment along with nutrition of the neonate. It is also generated by metabolic abnormalities that impact amelogenesis.

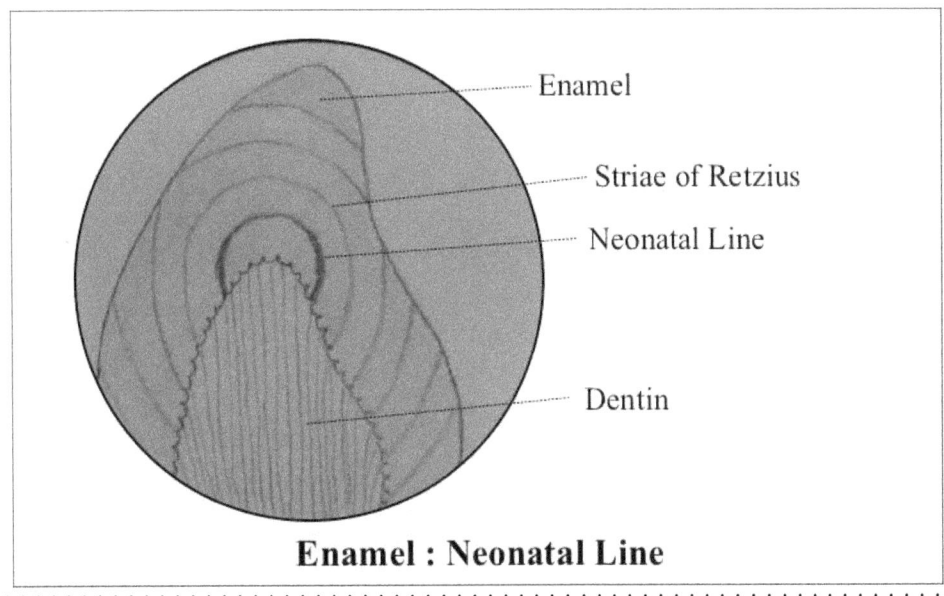

Enamel : Neonatal Line

****

Q7) Nasmyth's membrane

Q) Enamel cuticle.

Answer – *Enamel cuticle / Nasmyth's membrane,* is a fragile membrane that envelops the whole crown of a newly erupted tooth.

- This membrane, observed under an electron microscope, is a characteristic basal lamina located beneath any epithelium.
- It is the final substance secreted by ameloblasts upon the completion of enamel production.
- *Function* –It helps in the protection of mature enamel from the adjacent CT until the tooth emerges. Contact between CT and enamel may result in anomalies, such as enamel resorption or cementum deposition.
- Nasmyth's membrane is promptly eliminated by masticatory pressures. The enamel is later coated with pellicle, a deposit of salivary proteins.

****

Q8) Dentinoenamel junction.

Answer –The boundary between dentin and enamel is referred to as the dentinoenamel junction (DEJ).

- This junction is not linear; rather, it appears as a continuous scalloped line.
- At the DEJ, the dentin surface exhibits pitting, characterized by small depressions or concavities that accommodate the rounded projections of enamel. The enamel's convexities are oriented towards the dentin. This relationship will ensure that the firm retains enamel over dentin.
- The scalloped dentin-enamel junction is established prior to the development of enamel and dentin, as evidenced by the configuration of the ameloblasts.
- At the DEJ, mineral crystals of dentin and enamel intertwine.
- The DEJ is more prominent in the occlusal region where masticatory forces are high.

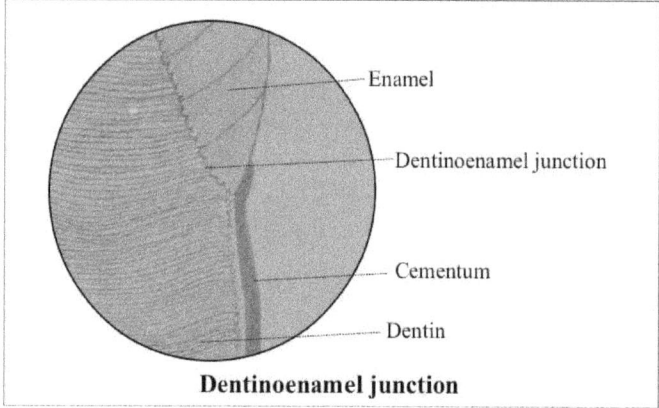

Dentinoenamel junction

****

Q9) Gnarled enamel.

Answer– The enamel rods are positioned perpendicular to the DEJ. In both the cervical region and the central areas of a deciduous tooth's crown, they are oriented horizontally. In the cervical area of the permanent tooth, the rods orient apically, whereas in the crown's central portion, they are horizontal.

- At incisal edge or cusp tip, bundles of enamel rods exhibit an uneven intertwining or twisting pattern. This visual phenomenon is referred to as *gnarled enamel*.

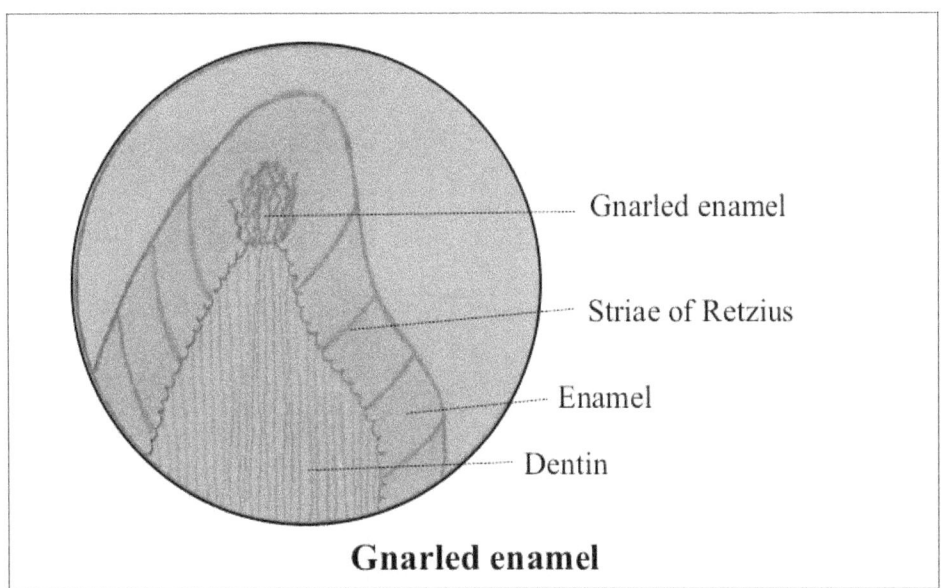

Gnarled enamel

***

Q10) Enamel spindle.

Answer –Odontoblastic processes from the dentin occasionally traverse the dentinoenamel junction. They are enlarged at its extremity. These are referred to as enamel spindles.

- They traverse perpendicularly to the DEJ.
- They are predominantly located in cusp tip region.
- In-ground section of teeth, organic material within the spindles decomposes and is substituted by air. Consequently, these air-filled cavities look dark under transmitted light.
- They are regions that are hypomineralized or partially mineralized. It possesses a lower concentration of calcium and phosphorus compared to enamel rods.

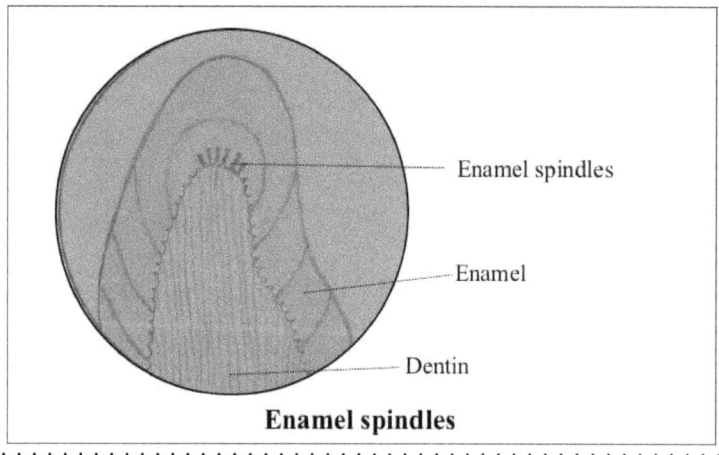
Enamel spindles

****

Q11) Perikymata.

Answer–Perikymata is transverse, wave-like grooves observed on surface of newly erupted teeth.

- They are considered to signify the outward appearance of striae of Retzius.
- They traverse the perimeter of the tooth surface.
- They are parallel to one another and the cementoenamel junction.
- *Number*--Their quantity is greater in the cervical region and diminishes towards the occlusal surface or incisal edge.
- Perikymata exhibit an almost consistent path. However, in the cervical region of the tooth, it may exhibit slight irregularities.

****

Q12) Ameloblast.

Answer – Ameloblasts are the cells that secrete enamel matrix.

Their formation occurs through the differentiation of inner enamel epithelial cells during the bell stage of tooth development.

The life span of ameloblasts can be divided into six stages.

- **Morphogenic stage** -- In the morphogenic stage, the IEE cells are characterized by a short or low columnar shape, possessing big oval nuclei that nearly occupy the entire cell body. The Golgi apparatus and centrioles are located in the proximal/basal end of the cell, namely the end adjacent to the SI, in contrast, the mitochondria are distributed uniformly throughout the cytoplasm.
- **Organizing stage** -- During the organizing phase, the IEE's cells (future ameloblasts) alter their morphology. They assume a tall, columnar form. Golgi bodies and centrioles migrate from proximal end of the cell to the distal end, i.e., the cell end which faces the dentin.

- **Formative stage** -- Upon the formation of the initial layer of dentin, there is transformation if IEE cells into ameloblasts. The ameloblasts maintain consistent length and configuration throughout the process of enamel matrix development. Ameloblasts form blunt cellular processes that penetrate the basal lamina and penetrate into the predentin.
- **Maturative stage** -- Enamel maturation (complete mineralization) commences once the majority of the enamel matrix thickness has developed in the occlusal or incisal region.
- **Protective stage** -- Upon complete deposition and calcification of the enamel, the ameloblasts are organized into a distinct layer. It is indistinguishable from the OEE and SI cells.
- The outer enamel epithelium, stratum intermedium, and ameloblast subsequently create a stratified epithelial layer over the enamel, referred to as *reduced enamel epithelium*.
- **Desmolytic stage** -- During the desmolytic phase, the REE undergoes proliferation and merges with the superficial oral epithelium. The cells at the core of this fused epithelium undergo degeneration due to insufficient nutrition, resulting in a perforation that facilitates tooth eruption.

****

Q13) Physical properties and chemical composition of enamel.

Answer –Enamel is the most resistant calcified tissue in body, giving a tooth's crown a layer of protection.

Physical properties:

Color--The color of enamel is determined by the extent of calcification and its uniformity. Teeth with a yellowish color possess transparent enamel. Grayish teeth possess opaque enamel.

Thickness – The enamel thickness differs across several regions of the tooth. The thickness measures 2 to 2.5 millimeters in the cusp region of molars and premolars and is nearly negligible at the cervical boundary of the tooth.

Hardness -- The body's most resilient calcified tissue is enamel. The hardness results from its elevated mineral content and crystalline structure. The enamel in permanent teeth is denser than that in deciduous teeth. The hardness is maximal at the surface and diminishes towards the DEJ. The denseness is maximal at the cusps and incisal ridges, diminishing towards the cervical line.

Brittleness– The composition and rigidity of enamel make it fragile, particularly when it deteriorates below a foundation of good dentin.

Permeability -- Enamel exhibits a considerable degree of permeability. It functions as a semipermeable membrane for certain ions and low molecular weight dyes. The outer layer of enamel is more permeable to saliva.

Chemical composition:

- By weight, enamel is made up of 4% organic matter and water and 96% inorganic stuff.
- The inorganic component primarily exists as hydroxyapatite crystals [$Ca_{10}(PO_4)_6(OH)_2$].

- Organic composition primarily consists of enamel proteins, comprising ninety percent amelogenins and ten percent non-amelogenins.
- *Hydroxyapatite crystals* -- Hydroxyapatite crystals exhibit a hexagonal cross-section. Each crystal possesses a center core of hydroxyl ions, around that calcium and phosphorus ions are organized. Magnesium can occasionally substitute for calcium, and carbonate can replace hydroxyl ions. The hydroxyapatite crystals within the enamel rods are oriented nearly parallel to rods longitudinal axis. These crystals deviate around 65 degrees from the principal axis as they extend toward the "tails" of the prisms.

****

Q14) Surface structures of enamel.

Answer – A rather amorphous layer of enamel is observed in seventy percent of permanent teeth and in all deciduous teeth. This is called *prismless (aprismatic) enamel* as it does not have a rod, rod sheath, and inter rod substance. It is soon lost by abrasion, attrition, and erosion.

Additional formations noted on the external enamel surface of newly erupted teeth include........

- **Rod ends** –On the enamel surface, the rod ends appear as concave pits of varied depths and shapes. In cervical region it is shallow, while in the incisal or occlusal surfaces they are deep.
- **Enamel cap**-- Small elevations are also seen on the enamel surface and are called *enamel caps*. These are due to the deposition of enamel on non-mineralized debris.
- **Pellicle** – Surface of newly erupted tooth is covered by pellicle. Upon contact with saliva, salivary proteins (mucins, glycoprotein's) bind to the tooth surface, resulting in the pellicle's formation.
- **Perikymata** - Refer to short notes Q11 in the chapter "Enamel."
- **Cracks**– Refer to short notes Q18 in chapter "Enamel".

****

Q15) Age changes in enamel.

Answer –*The following changes are noted in enamel with ageing.....*

1] Attrition or degradation of the occlusal surface and the proximal contact areas. This is attributed to masticatory pressures.

2] A localized elevation of specific elements (e.g., nitrogen, fluorine, etc.) is observed in the superficial enamel layers of aged teeth.

3] The teeth may become darker with ageing. This can be attributed to alterations in the organic composition of the enamel at the surface. Consequently, resistance to deterioration is enhanced with age.

4] There is reduced permeability to fluids in older teeth. This may result from the enlargement of the hydroxyapatite crystals.

****

Q16) Ultrastructure of enamel.

Answer – Ultrastructure of enamel is studied under electron microscope. Following are the features that can be seen.

- *Enamel rods* -- Human enamel consists of structural units known as enamel rods, which are encased in a rod sheath and divided by interrod material. The enamel rods are commonly arranged in a keyhole or paddle-shaped prism configuration. Longitudinal sections traverse the "heads" or "bodies" of one row of rods and the "tails" of an adjacent row. This creates the illusion of rods being divided by interrod material. The rods "tails" face cervically, while their "bodies" are orientated toward the occlusal or incisal surfaces. The hydroxyapatite crystalsare nearly parallel to the rods long axis, and these crystals deviate by about 65 degrees as they stretch into the prisms' "tails."
- *Aprismatic enamel*-- A rather amorphous layer of enamel is observed in seventy percent of permanent teeth and in all deciduous teeth. This is called *prismless/aprismatic enamel* as it does not have rod, rod sheath and inter rod substance. It is soon lost by abrasion, attrition, and erosion.
- *Rod ends and enamel caps* -- On the enamel surface, the rod ends appear as concave pits of varied depths and shapes. They are shallow in cervical region, while at the incisal or occlusal surfaces they are deep. Minor protrusions are also observed on the enamel surface, referred to as *enamel caps*. These result from the deposition of enamel on non-mineralized debris.

****

Q17) Reduced enamel epithelium.

Answer –Upon complete deposition and calcification of the enamel, the ameloblasts responsible for its formation will organize into a distinct layer. They lose their tall columnar configuration and acquire a cuboidal form. They can no longer be distinguished from the OEE and SI cells. On the surface of the newly formed enamel, the OEE, SI and ameloblast cells form a stratified epithelial layer known as REE.

Function of reduced enamel epithelium–Until the tooth erupts, REE shields the new enamel from the surrounding connective tissue. Contact between CT and enamel may result in anomalies, such as enamel resorption or cementum deposition.

****

Q18) Enamel cracks.

Answer — Enamel cracks are slender fissure-like formations observed on the external surface of nearly all teeth. Enamel cracks signify the peripheral boundaries of the enamel lamellae, similar to perikymata, which denote the external manifestation of striae of Retzius.

Most of them are less than a millimeter in length. They extend for varying distances on the surface perpendicular to the DEJ.

Q19) Incremental lines in the hard tissues of the tooth.

Answer —Incremental lines in the dental hard tissues are…..

Incremental lines in enamel

Striae of Retzius – Refer to short notes Q5 in chapter 'Enamel'.

Neonatal line in enamel -- The deciduous teeth's enamel forms both prenatally and postnatally. The demarcation between pre- and post-natal enamel is shown by a distinct incremental line of Retzius referred to as the neonatal line or ring. The darkening of the striae of Retzius seems to occur from abrupt alterations in the environment and nutrition of the neonate.

Incremental lines in dentin

Lines of von Ebner –Refer to short notes Q4 in chapter 'Dentin'.

Contour lines of Owen -- Certain incremental lines are darker and are referred to as Owen's *contour lines*. This is attributable to disruptions in the matrix formation and mineralization processes. It is most effectively observed in longitudinal ground sections. These are classified as hypocalcified bands.

Neonatal line in dentin -- Dentin in deciduous teeth forms partially before birth (prenatal dentin) and partially after birth (postnatal dentin). The demarcation between pre-natal and post-natal dentin is shown by a distinct incremental line which is called the neonatal line or ring. The darkening of the increment seems to arise from abrupt changes in environment and nourishment of newborn infants.

Incremental lines in cementum

Lines of Salter -- Refer to short notes Q6 in chapter 'Cementum'.

Q20) Incremental lines.

Answer — Refer to short notes Q19 in chapter "Enamel".

Incremental lines in bone – Refer to short notes Q1 in chapter "Bone".

DENTIN

MAIN QUESTIONS

Q1) Discuss in detail about the various types of dentin. Add a note on its physical properties.

Answer -- The major mass of the tooth, which gives it its overall structure, is made up of specialized calcified connective tissue called dentin.

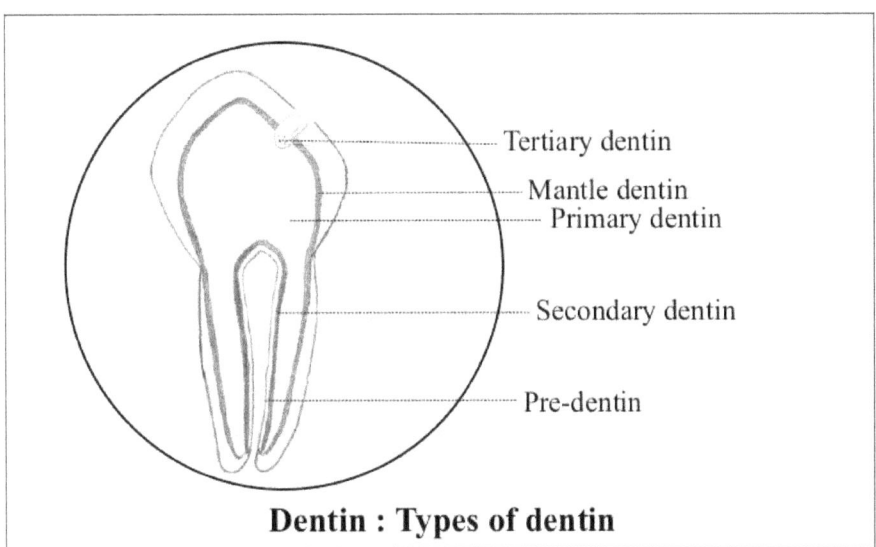

Dentin : Types of dentin

TYPES OF DENTIN

1] Primary dentin ---- Mantle dentin

---- Circumpulpal dentin

2] Secondary dentin

3] Tertiary dentin

PRIMARY DENTIN

Primary dentin is the initially developed dentin. It is established prior to root completion or until the tooth attains functionality.

Types

There are two kinds of it. ----- Mantle dentin

Circumpulpal dentin

Mantle dentin

✓ Mantle dentin is the initial dentin developed in the crown and is located directly under the

DEJ.
- ✓ It is the primary dentin's outermost or periphery.
- ✓ This area is flexible and offers a cushioning effect on the tooth.
- ✓ The organic matrix has large collagen fibers oriented at right angle to the DEJ.
- ✓ In comparison to circumpulpal dentin, which encases the pulp, mantle dentin exhibits lower mineralization and a reduced number of irregularities. Globular mineralization occurs in mantle dentin.

Circumpulpal dentin

- ✓ The dentin that surrounds the pulp and constitutes the primary mass of the tooth is the circumpulpal dentin.
- ✓ It has smaller-sized, closely packed collagen fibers compared to mantle dentin.
- ✓ Mineralization is by globular or linear pattern. It may possess a higher mineral content than the mantle dentin.

SECONDARY DENTIN

- ✓ It is developed after primary dentin.
- ✓ It is deposited following root completion.
- ✓ It is a thin dentin band next to the pulp.
- ✓ It accumulates at a diminished rate throughout an individual's lifetime.
- ✓ The pulp chamber has its increased thickness on the roof and floor.
- ✓ It contains fewer tubules which are less regular compared to primary dentin. Tubules are continuing with those of primary dentin. Bend in the tubules is seen at junction between primary and secondary dentin (SD).
- ✓ Its organic and inorganic content is similar to primary dentin.

TERTIARY DENTIN

Synonyms -- Reactionary or reparative dentin.

- ✓ The localized production of dentin at pulp-dentin interface, triggered by stimuli like as trauma from caries, restorative operations, attrition, abrasion or erosion is referred to as tertiary dentin.
- ✓ It is developed only at certain locations by odontoblasts in response to stimuli.
- ✓ The pace of deposition is dependent upon the severity of the injury; the more severe the trauma, the more accelerated is the deposition rate.
- ✓ The composition of tertiary dentin is contingent upon the intensity along with duration of stimulation. It may possess tubules that are continuous with those of SD, or it may have fewer tubules that are unevenly distributed, or sometimes it may lack tubules entirely. Odontoblasts may at time be captured within the speedily deposited dentin (osteodentin).

- ✓ Existing odontoblasts respond to a modest stimulus by producing reactionary dentin. In case of severe intensity stimulus, the odontoblasts are killed. New odontoblasts differentiate from cells in the cell-rich zone of pulp and produce tertiary dentin.

  'Physical properties of dentin' refer to section 'Physical properties' in short notes Q1in chapter 'Dentin'.

  ****

Q2) Discuss in detail dentinogenesis.

Answer – The tooth's basic mass and general shape are provided by the specialized calcified connective tissue known as dentin. The process of dentin formation is known as dentinogenesis.

- ✓ Dentin formation continues throughout the life span of an individual.
- ✓ Dentinogenesis begins during bell stage of odontogenesis. It begins at the concave apex of the folded IEE, the area allocated for the future cusp tip or incisal edge, and thereafter extends down the cuspal slope.
- ✓ Dentin formation in teeth with many cusps initiates independently at each prospective cusp tip and gradually extends down the cuspal slope until it merges with neighboring formative centers.
- ✓ The organ responsible for dentin production is the "dental papilla. Under the influence of the inner enamel epithelial cells, the odontoblasts, the cells that produce dentin, differentiate from the ectomesenchymal cells of the dental papilla.

ODONTOBLAST DIFFERENTIATION
- ✓ Odontoblasts are the cells that secrete the collagen fibers and other extracellular matrix components of dentin.
- ✓ Signal from the IEE cells initiates differentiation of odontoblasts from the undifferentiated mesenchymal cells of the dental papilla. They undergo mitotic division to produce an odontoblast and another daughter cell that persists as a subodontoblast cell.
- ✓ Odontoblasts generate processes, known as odontoblastic processes, which remain embedded within the developing extracellular dentin matrix as it advances towards the pulp.

Dentinogenesis is a two-phase process
- ✓ *Phase 1*: In the first phase there is formation of organic matrix (called predentin)
- ✓ *Phase 2*: In this phase, there is calcification of the formed dentinal matrix.
- ✓ A layer of predentin forms at the pulp edge and persists for one day before undergoing mineralization. Once it mineralizes, a new layer of predentin is formed.

MINERALIZATION
Two types of dentin mineralization are seen in histology.

- ✓ <u>Mineralization as linear deposits (linear mineralization)</u> -- Within the ground substance and on the surface of the collagen fibrils, hydroxyapatite crystals are deposited in this pattern of dentin mineralization.

- ✓ Mineralization by fusion of globules (globular mineralization) -- In this pattern of dentin mineralization, several discrete globules/islands containing mineral crystals is deposited within the organic matrix. As crystal formation persists, the globular mass increases in size and ultimately fuses into a singular calcified entity. This pattern is observed in the mantle dentin's mineralization. In circumpulpal dentin, mineralization occurs in either a globular or linear form.

Formation of root dentin
- ✓ The development of root dentin occurs at a reduced pace after the formation of crown.
- ✓ The cells of "Hertwig's epithelial root sheath" (HERS) "stimulates the development of odontoblasts from the peripheral cells of the dental papilla in the root. These odontoblasts then secrete the root dentin.
- ✓ The mineralization level of root dentin differs from that of coronal dentin.

Secondary dentinogenesis
- ✓ SD is formed after completion of root development.
- ✓ The odontoblasts that generate primary dentin are also the ones that produce it.
- ✓ Deposition of primary and secondary dentin is in continuum.

Tertiary dentinogenesis
- ✓ In response to a mild stimulus, existing odontoblasts within the pulp create reactionary dentin. In instances of intense stimuli, the odontoblasts are destroyed. New odontoblasts arise from cells in the cell-rich zone of the pulp and synthesize tertiary dentin.

****

Q3) Write the physical properties and chemical composition of dentin. Describe the histology of dentinal tubules.

Answer –

Refer short notes Q1 for 'Physical and chemical properties of dentin' in chapter 'Dentin'.

Refer to section 'Dentinal tubules' in main question Q5 of chapter 'Dentin'.

****

Q4) Write the physical properties and chemical composition of dentin. Describe the various hypocalcified structures of dentin.

Answer –

Refer to 'Physical and chemical properties' in short notes Q1 of chapter 'Dentin'.

Refer to 'Hypocalcified areas in dentin' short notes Q19 in chapter 'Dentin'.

****

Q5) Describe in detail the microscopic structure of dentin.

Answer – The bulk of a tooth is made up of dentin, a specialized calcified connective tissue that gives the tooth its general structure. Various features are seen in dentin under a light microscope. For example,

- Dentinal tubules.
- Peritubular / Intratubular dentin.
- Intertubular dentin.
- Predentin.
- Incremental lines.
- Interglobular dentin.
- Tome's granular layer.
- Sclerotic dentin.
- Dead tracts.

DENTINAL TUBULES

- Dentinal tubules are characteristic of dentin. They are tubes within the dentin that extend from the pulp to dentinoenamel / dentinocemental junction. Each tubule houses an odontoblast process that finally terminates at the enamel or cementum junction.

- The arrangement of the dentinal tubule reflects the path followed by the odontoblast during dentinogenesis.

Course of dentinal tubules

- Dentinal tubules are perpendicular to dentinoenamel junction and dentinocemental junction.
- They have a gentle curve (resembling an "S" shape) in the crown. The curvature originates from the aggregation of odontoblasts as they migrate towards the pulp. The primary curvature begins at right angle to the pulpal surface, with the initial curve (or convexity) directed towards the root apex. In root dentin due to little or no crowding of the odontoblasts, the tubules take a straight course. It is straight near the incisal edge, cusp tip, and root tip. Secondary curvatures are also present along the entire course of the tubule.
- The tubules are elongated due to their S-shape, exceeding the thickness of the dentin.
- The crown contains a greater number of tubules than the root.
- Number of tubules on the pulpal side is more than on surface.
- The tubules have a tapered structure being larger at the pulpal surface and narrow at the DEJ.
- Tubules have lateral branches called *canaliculi / microtubules*. Odontoblastic processes in the dentinal tubules communicate with one another through these canaliculi. These lateral branches are more numerous in the root than in the crown.

- Certain odontoblastic processes penetrate the DEJ into the enamel for many millimeters, and are known as *enamel spindles*.

Occasionally, the odontoblastic process within the dentinal tubule may degenerate because of caries, attrition or abrasion, resulting in unfilled dentinal tubules filled with air. These are referred to as *dead tracts*. Dead tracts in reflected light appear white and in transmitted light black.

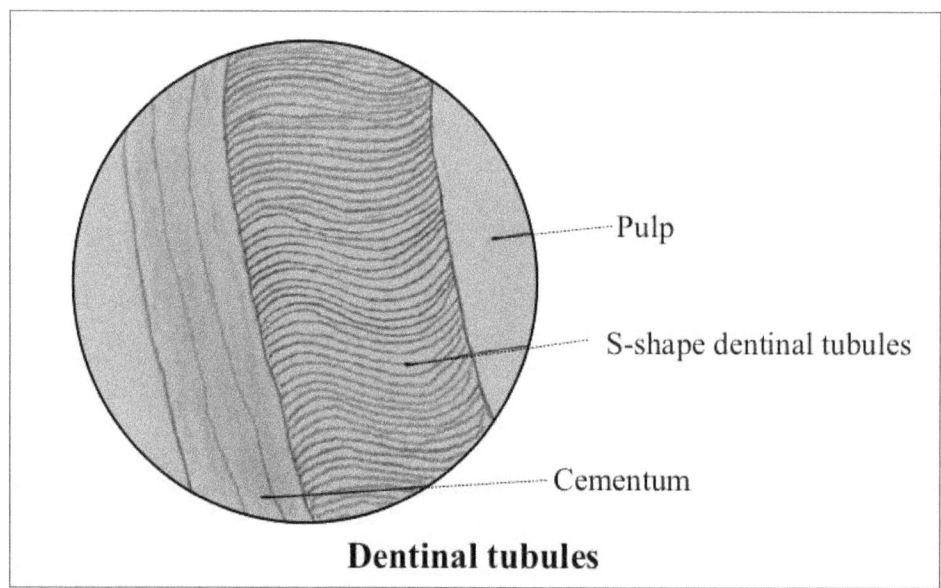

Dentinal tubules

Peritubular / Intratubular dentine

- The dentin directly surrounding the dentinal tubule producing a wall around each tubule is the peritubular or intratubular dentin.
- Compared to intertubular dentin, it is more mineralized.
- A space exists between the peritubular dentin and the odontoblastic process (periodontoblastic space) that holds dentinal fluid.

Intertubular dentine

- The dentin that is in between the dentinal tubules is referred to as intertubular dentin.
- It constitutes the primary mass of dentin.
- It is highly mineralized but less than peritubular dentin.

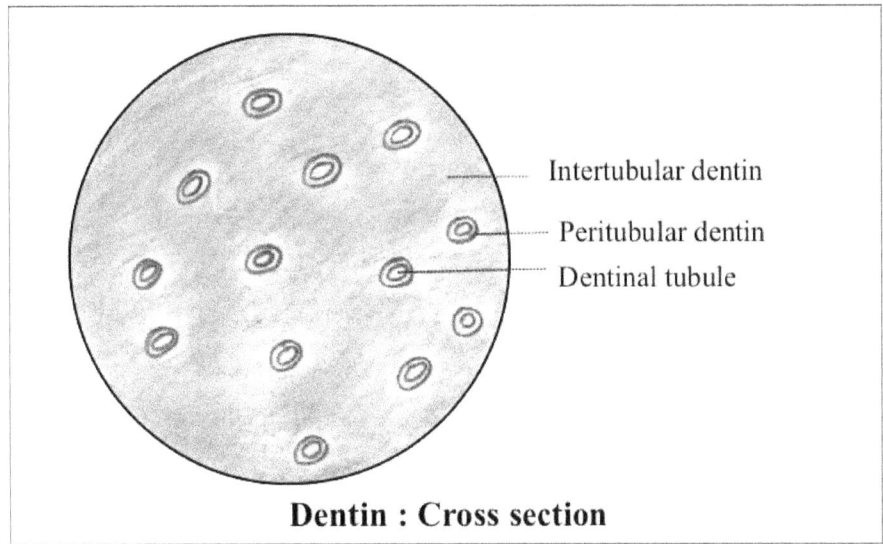

Dentin : Cross section

PREDENTIN

- It is located next to the pulp tissue and is unmineralized.
- It takes a lighter stain than the mineralized dentin due to the variation in the composition.
- A new layer of predentin is deposited when pre existing predentin changes into dentin due to mineralization at the predentin-dentin junction.

INCREMENTAL LINES

- ***Incremental lines of von Ebner*** -- Incremental lines of dentin are known as *lines of von Ebner*. They appear as slender lines within the dentin, oriented perpendicularly to the dentinal tubules. The incremental lines signify the typical daily rhythmic and linear pattern of dentin deposition. It is readily observable in ground sections.

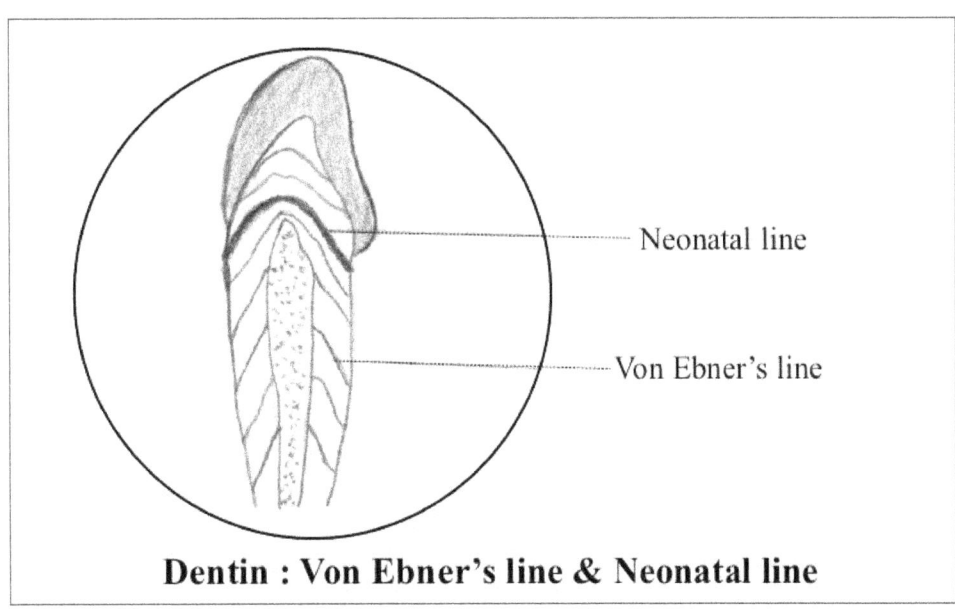

Dentin : Von Ebner's line & Neonatal line

- ***Contour lines of Owen***—Certain incremental lines are darker and are referred to as *contour lines of Owen*. This is attributable to disruptions in the matrix formation and mineralization processes. It is best seen in longitudinal ground sections. These are considered hypocalcified bands.
- ***Neonatal line*** -- The dentin in deciduous teeth forms partially before birth (prenatal dentin) and partially after birth (postnatal dentin). The demarcation between pre- and postnatal dentin is shown by a distinct incremental line known as the neonatal line or ring. The darkening of the incremental seems to occur from abrupt changes in the newborn infant's environment and nourishment.

INTERGLOBULAR DENTIN

- In globular mineralization pattern, discrete globules/islands containing mineral crystals are deposited within the organic matrix of dentin. As crystal formation persists, the globular mass increases in size and ultimately combines into a singular calcified entity.
- Failure of fusion of these globular masses results in *interglobular dentin*.
- It represents a hypomineralized area.
- The appearance of dentinal tubules within the interglobular dentin signifies a mineralization problem rather than a matrix formation issue.
- It is typically observed in the circumpulpal dentin, situated just beneath the mantle dentin.
- It usually affects the middle and cervical thirds of the root and crown.
- It appears black in ground sections.

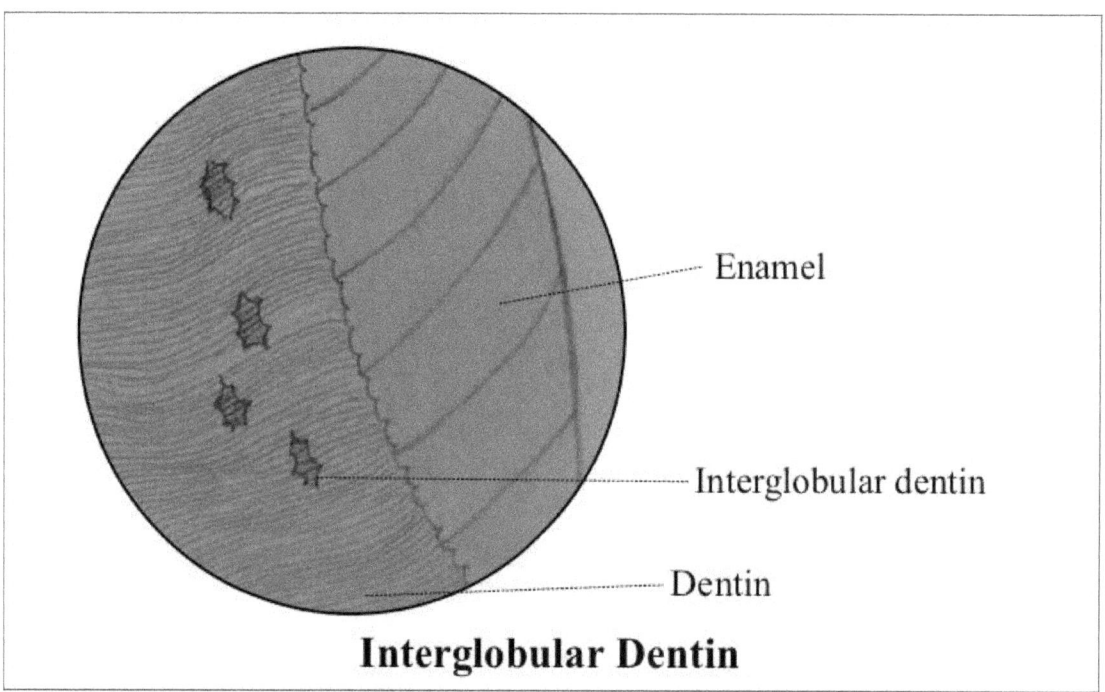

Interglobular Dentin

TOMES GRANULAR LAYER

- Root dentin when seen under transmitted light in ground section, a granular area known as Tomes granular layer is seen just adjacent to the cementum. The granular texture of this layer is believed to result from the fusion and looping of terminal segments of dentinal tubules.
- It is a hypomineralized area.
- This zone progressively widens from the CEJ to the root apex.

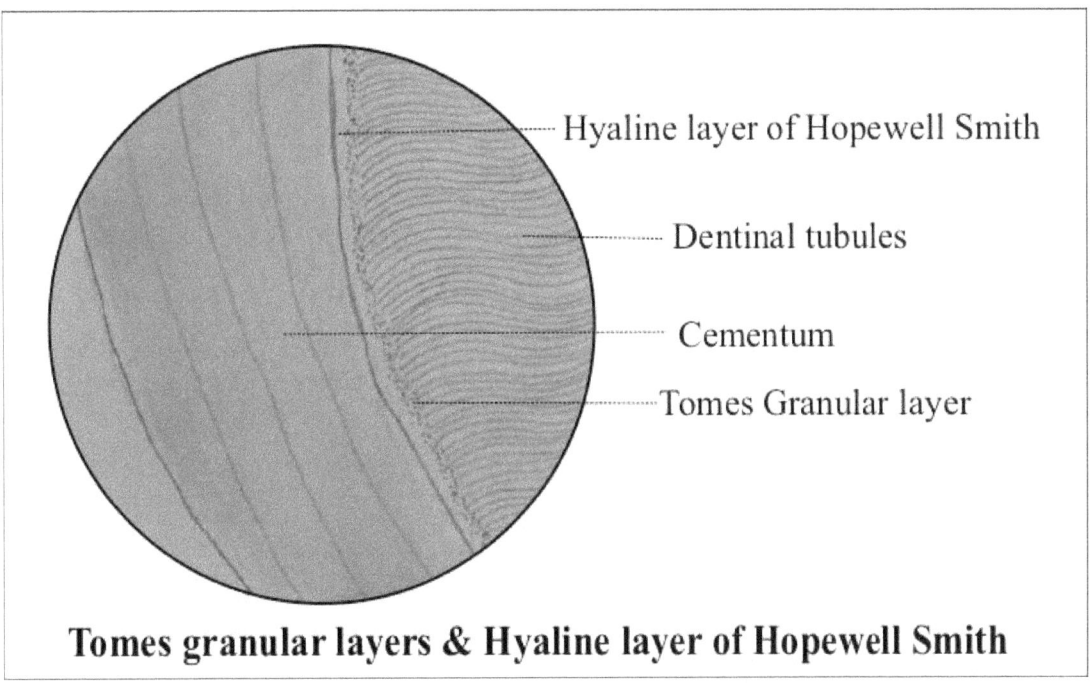

Tomes granular layers & Hyaline layer of Hopewell Smith

SCLEROTIC DENTIN

- Sclerotic/transparent dentin refers to dentinal tubules that have been occluded with calcified substances. The dentinal tubules get blocked as a result of persistent mineral deposition in peritubular dentin.
- Sclerotic dentin in ground sections exhibits a transparent or glassy appearance under transmitted light and appears dark under reflected light.
- *Site* - apical part of the root and between the pulp surface and the DEJ in the crown.
- *Age* – seen in old age. The amount increases with ageing. It is considered a normal physiologic defensive response of dentin to protect the pulp.

DEAD TRACTS

- Odontoblastic process in the dentinal tubule may die leaving behind empty dentinal tubules filled with air. These are known as *dead tracts*.
- Loss of odontoblastic process may be due to caries, attrition, abrasion, etc.
- Dead tracts in reflected light appear white and in transmitted light black.

- Dead tract areas show decreased sensitivity.
- They are common in older age groups.

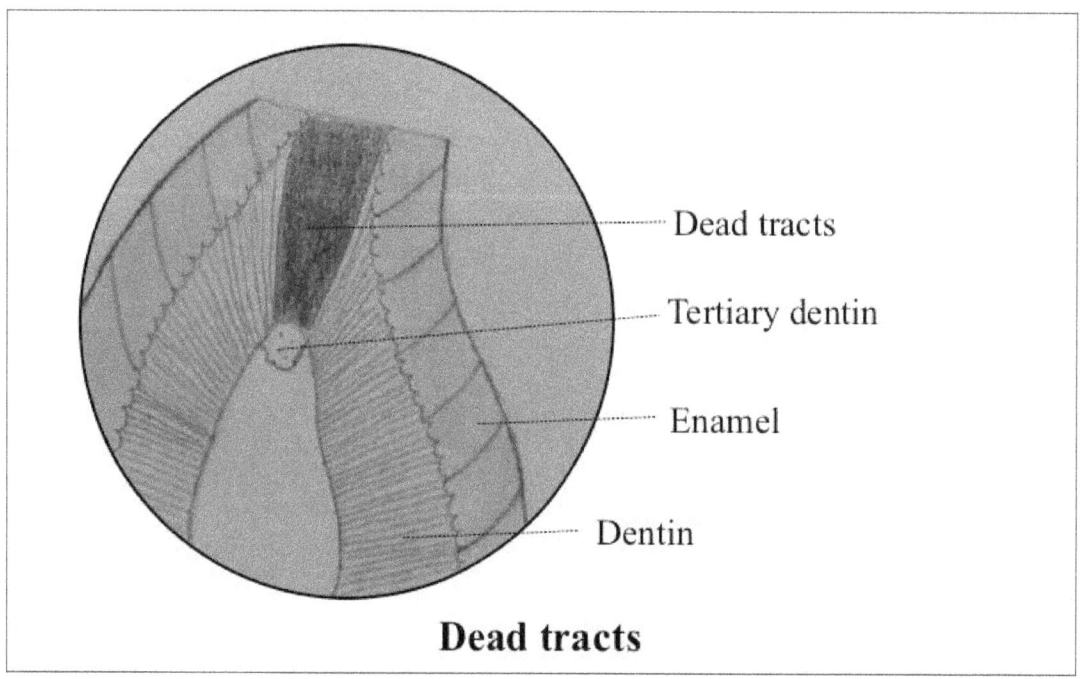

Dead tracts

....

SHORT NOTES

Q1) Physical and chemical properties of dentin.

Answer -- The basic mass of the tooth and the component that gives it its overall shape is dentin, a specialized calcified connective tissue.

Physical Properties of Dentin:

Colour–Dentin is pale yellow and darkens with age.

Hardness -- Dentin is less rigid and fragile compared to enamel. The center is stronger than the periphery or the vicinity of the pulp. It is denser than bone but less dense than enamel. The hardness of dentin in primary teeth is lower than that in permanent teeth.

Elasticity –It possesses viscoelastic properties and is susceptible to little deformation. The elasticity of dentin prevents the fracturing of the overlying fragile enamel.

Permeability –Dentin is semi-permeable. Permeability decreases with age.

Chemical composition of dentin

- ✓ 35% of dentin is organic and the other 65% is inorganic.
- ✓ Inorganic content contains "Hydroxyapatite crystals" [$Ca_{10}(PO_4)_6(OH)_2$].

✓ The organic composition consists primarily of collagen fibers (90% type I with minor proportions of type III and type V), 10% water and non-collagenous matrix proteins, including dentin phosphoprotein, dentin glycoprotein, dentin sialoprotein, dentin matrix protein-1 and osteonectin, along with trace amounts of phosphates, carbonates, and sulfates.

****

Q2) Dentinal tubules.

Answer-- Refer to section 'Dentinal tubules' in main question Q5 of chapter 'Dentin'.

****

Q3) Curvatures in dentinal tubules.

Answer -- Refer to section 'Dentinal tubules' in main question Q5 of chapter 'Dentin'.

****

Q4) Incremental lines in dentin.

Answer -- Refer to section 'Incremental lines' in main question Q5 of chapter 'Dentin'.

****

Q5) Structural lines in dentin.

Answer -- Refer to section 'Incremental lines' in main question Q5 of chapter 'Dentin'.

****

Q6) Intratubular / Peritubular dentin.

Answer-- Refer to section 'Intratubular / Peritubular dentin' in main question Q5 of chapter 'Dentin'.

****

Q7) Interglobular dentin.

Answer-- Refer to section 'Interglobular dentin' in main question Q5 of chapter 'Dentin'.

****

Q8) Primary, secondary, and tertiary dentin.

Answer -- Refer to section 'Types of dentin' in main question Q1 of chapter 'Dentin'.

****

Q9) Tertiary dentin / Reparative dentin.

Answer -- Refer to section 'Tertiary dentin' in main question Q1 of chapter 'Dentin'.

****

Q10) Dentinogenesis.

Answer -- Refer to main question Q2 of chapter 'Dentin'.

****

Q11) Theories of dentin sensitivity

Q) Dentin sensitivity theories.

Answer – Dentin hypersensitivity is characterized by acute, transient discomfort originating from exposed dentin in reaction to many stimuli, including thermal, evaporative, chemical, tactile and osmotic factors.

There are three theories to describe dentin sensitivity.

Direct neural stimulation theory

- According to this theory pain or sensitivity is transmitted by direct stimulation of the nerves present in dentin.
- The nerves in dentin are limited only to inner dentin and are not easily seen.
- The concept was rejected due to the ineffectiveness of topical local anesthetics in diminishing sensitivity.

Hydrodynamic / Fluid theory

- This is the most popular theory.
- This theory suggests that stimuli such as heat and cold influence fluid dynamics within the dentinal tubule. Fluid movement, whether inward or outward, in the dentinal tubule, induces mechanical disruption of the neurons associated with the odontoblast or its processes. Consequently, these neurons function as mechanoreceptors to convey pain or dentinal sensitivity.
- Evidence was available in support of this theory. On exposed dentin surface blebs of fluid could be seen. Drying this region with air or cotton results in increased fluid loss and heightened pain. The heightened sensitivity at the DEJ results from the branching of nerve terminals in that area.

Transduction theory

- This theory is of the opion that the process of odontoblast present within the dentinal tubules transmitted pain stimuli to nerve endings located in predentin, odontoblast zone and pulp.
- This theory was not accepted as the odontoblast process had no neurotransmitter vesicles which are necessary for pain transmission.

****

Q12) Hydrodynamic theory of dentin sensitivity.

Answer -- Refer to section 'Hydrodynamic theory' in short notes Q11 of chapter 'Dentin'.

****

Q13) Dead tracts.

Answer --Refer to section 'Dead tracts' in main question Q5 of chapter 'Dentin'.

****

Q14) Sclerotic dentin

Q) Transparent dentin.

Answer -- Refer section 'Sclerotic dentin / Transparent dentin' in main question Q5 of chapter 'Dentin'.

****

Q15) Age changes in dentin.

Answer–With ageing, the thickness of dentin increases due to progressive dentin deposition. The other changes that take place are

a) Reparative dentin.
b) Sclerotic dentin.
c) Dead tracts

Refer to sections 'Reparative dentin,' 'Sclerotic dentin,' 'Dead tracts' in main question Q5 of chapter 'Dentin'.

****

Q16) Enumerate different types of dentin and write about interglobular dentin.

Answer --

Refer to section 'types of dentin' in main question Q1 of chapter 'Dentin'.

Refer to section 'Interglobular dentin' in main question Q5 of chapter 'Dentin'.

****

Q17) Tome's granular layer.

Answer --Refer to section 'Tomes granular layer' in main question Q5 of chapter 'Dentin'.

****

Q18) Structures of dentin.

Answer -- Refer to main question Q5 of chapter 'Dentin'.

****

Q19) Hypocalcified areas/structures in dentin.

Answer – Hypocalcified areas in dentin are

a) Incremental lines (lines of von Ebner, contour lines of Owen, neonatal line).
b) Interglobular dentin.
c) Tome's granular layer.

Refer to sections 'Incremental lines,' 'Interglobular dentin,' and 'Tomes granular layer' in main question Q5 of chapter 'Dentin'.

****

DENTAL PULP

MAIN QUESTIONS

Q1) Describe the histology of dental pulp.

Answer – *The tooth's pulp chamber and root canals contain dental pulp, a soft, specialized connective tissue that is highly vascularized and innervated.*

Four clear-cut zones can be seen in the histology of dental pulp…….

- *Odontoblastic zone*
- *Cell-free zone of Weil*
- *Cell-rich zone*
- *Pulp core*

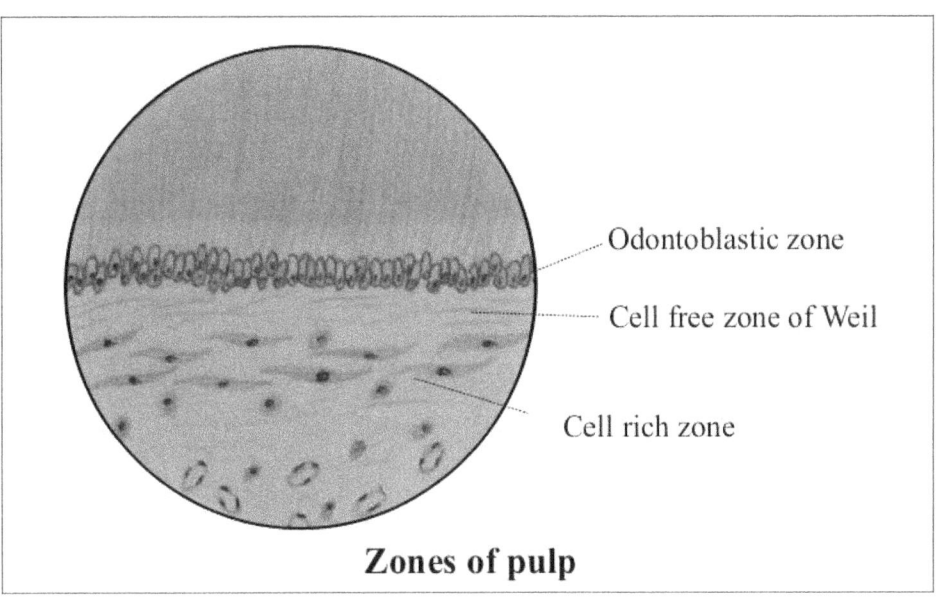

Zones of pulp

ODONTOBLASTIC ZONE

- Odontoblastic zone is the outermost zone of pulp.
- This region consists of odontoblasts that create a layer at the perimeter of the pulp. It is the pulp's second-most prominent cell after fibroblasts.
- Shape and organelle content of odontoblasts vary depending upon their functional activity. Active cells possess elongated columnar body with prominent oval nuclei located in the basal region of the cell. Abundant rER, Golgi apparatus and many mitochondria are located next to the nucleus. Inactive cells are small, possessing minimal cytoplasm and a reduced quantity of organelles.

- Odontoblasts have a tall columnar body in crown, a cuboidal form in the mid-root region and an ovoid to spindle shape at the root apex. They are in close proximity to one another and are connected by junctional complexes.

CELL-FREE ZONE OF WEIL

- This second layer of pulp is present beneath the odontoblastic zone.
- It is prevalent in coronal pulp and typically absent in radicular pulp.
- It is an area where odontoblasts migrate towards the pulp during tooth growth.
- It does not contain cells but has processes of fibroblasts, nerves, axons and capillaries.
- It is suggested to be an artifact (false appearance) produced during histological processing and caused due to the shrinkage of odontoblasts and the deeper pulp tissue.

CELL-RICH ZONE

- A cell-rich zone is located adjacent to a cell-free zone.
- In the coronal pulp, it is eminent.
- This layer predominantly contains fibroblasts and undifferentiated mesenchymal cells.
- The zone has a rich network of capillaries and nerve axons.

Fibroblasts

- These are the most abundant cells in the pulp after odontoblasts.
- They are sizable, spindle-shaped cells characterized by ample cytoplasm and multiple organelles involved in protein synthesis and secretion, including rER, Golgi apparatus, secretory vesicles, along with mitochondria.
- They are aligned with the fiber bundles. They possess elongated, slender cytoplasmic extensions that encircle these fiber bundles.
- Fibroblasts contact each other by their processes and adhere to each other by cell junctions.
- In aged pulp they appear round/spindle-shaped and have short processes with few organelles (now called *fibrocytes*).
- If fibroblast function is affected, there is decreased fiber synthesis leading to the loss of tooth's supporting tissue.

Undifferentiated mesenchymal cells

- Refer to short notes Q7 in chapter 'Pulp'.

PULP CORE

- The pulp core is located at the tooth's center.
- It is similar to the connective tissue found in other sites.
- It consists of major blood vessels, nerves and lymphatic channels.

Defense cells

▶ The immune cells consist of histiocytes, macrophages, mast cells and plasma cells.

▶ In addition to these cells, there are several vascular components, including neutrophils, eosinophils, basophils, lymphocytes, along with monocytes. These cells move from the pulp's blood arteries and responds to inflammation.

Blood supply

▶ Pulp is highly vascularized. Minor arteries and arterioles penetrate the apical foramen and proceed directly to the coronal pulp. As it moves through the radicular pulp, it produces a number of branches which pass outwards to form a plexus in the odontogenic region.

Nerve supply

▶ Nerves penetrate the pulp via apical foramen along side blood vessels. They split to create a plexus in the acellular region of pulp, situated under the odontoblastic zone in the crown of the tooth (*subodontoblastic plexus of Raschkow*). Nerve axons from this plexus traverse the cell-dense and acellular zones of the pulp. They either end adjacent to the odontoblast layer or traverse along side the process of odontoblast within the dentinal tubules.

Extracellular substance

▶ It is gel-like in nature.
▶ It consists of acid mucopolysaccharides and protein polysaccharides.

****

SHORT NOTES

Q1) Pulp stones

Q) Denticles.

Answer– These are also called *'pulp stones'* or *'denticles'*.

▶ Nodular calcified masses are observed in the coronal and radicular pulp, with a higher prevalence in the coronal pulp.
▶ They may be single or multiple in a tooth.
▶ They are typically asymptomatic unless they exert pressure on nerves and blood vessels.
▶ It is seen in both functional and also in unerupted teeth.
▶ They expand in size by gradual deposition of minerals on its surface.
▶ The incidence of their occurrence increases with age.
▶ *Significance–* Its presence decreases the quantity of pulpal cells. It obstructs the cleansing and expansion of the root canal during endodontic therapy.

Types of pulp stones

a) True pulp stones and false pulp stones.

b) Free, attached and embedded pulp stones.

True pulp stones

- True pulp stones have a structure similar to dentin i.e. they have dentinal tubules that contain odontoblastic process.
- *Site*–These are seen close to apical foramen.
- *Cause* – The inclusion of epithelial root sheath cells within the pulp is hypothesized to stimulate pulp cells to develop into odontoblasts, subsequently leading to dentin formation.

False pulp stones

- False pulp stones lack dentinal tubules and odontoblastic processes.
- They appear as concentric layers of calcified mass.
- The centre of false pulp stones may contain necrotic debris and calcified mass.

Free pulp stones –The pulp stones are freely situated within the pulp and fully enclosed by the pulp tissue.

Attached pulp stones – The pulp stones are partially fused or connected to the adjacent dentin.

Embedded pulp stones– These pulp stones are completely enclosed within dentin. Initially, these pulp stones may be lying free in the pulpal tissue. As dentin is deposited throughout life, they may initially get attached to this dentin being deposited (attached pulp stone) and later on gets embedded into it (embedded pulp stone).

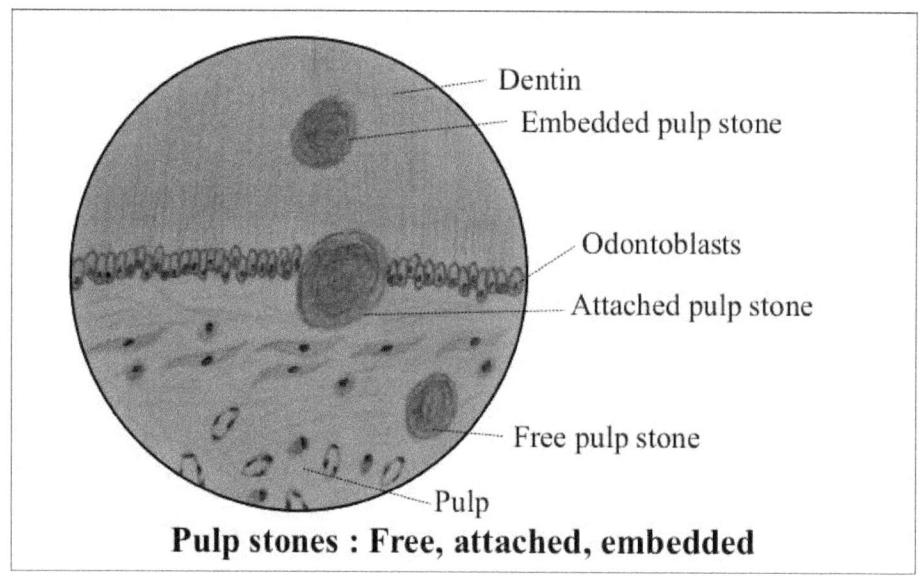

Pulp stones : Free, attached, embedded

Diffuse or linear calcifications

▸ These are irregular calcified deposits seen in the pulp tissue.
▸ *Site* – Common in radicular pulp and rare in coronal pulp.
▸ They are typically observed in near collagen fiber bundles or blood vessels.
▸ Coronal pulp may be normal without any inflammation even in the presence of linear calcifications in the root canal.

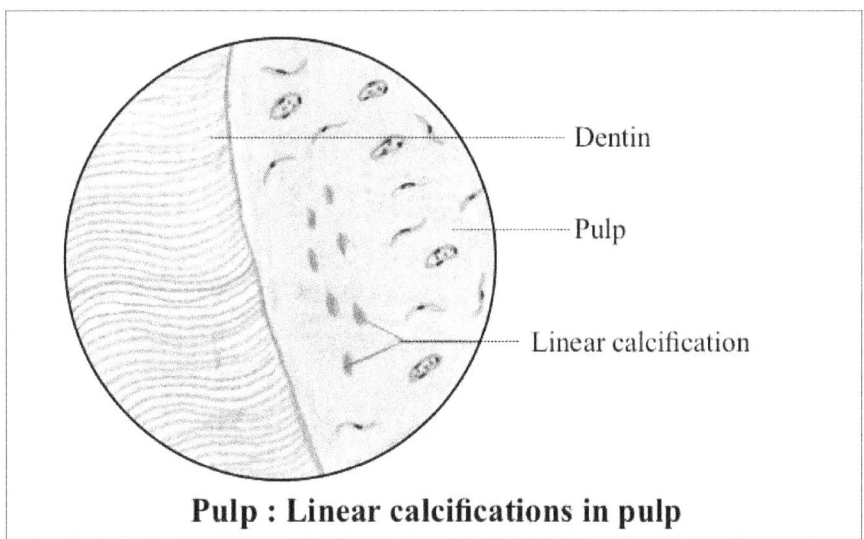

Pulp : Linear calcifications in pulp

****

Q2) Accessory canals.

Answer – Accessory canals are additional channels that run laterally from the root pulp, traversing the root dentin into the periodontal ligament (PDL). It can be observed along the whole length of the root, though it is more prevalent in the apical third.

Clinical significance

▸ Accessory canals serve as channels for the transmission of infection from pulp to PDL or vice versa.

Mechanism of formation

▸ The exact mechanism of its formation is unclear.
▸ The root sheath cells stimulate the odontoblast's differentiation from the dental papilla cells, which subsequently generate dentin. In premature loss of root sheath cells, there is no differentiation of odontoblasts and thus no dentin is formed, thereby leading to a track formation (accessory canal).
▸ It may also be seen in locations where the growing root crosses a blood artery. The hard tissue may be deposited around the blood vessel, thereby making a lateral canal.

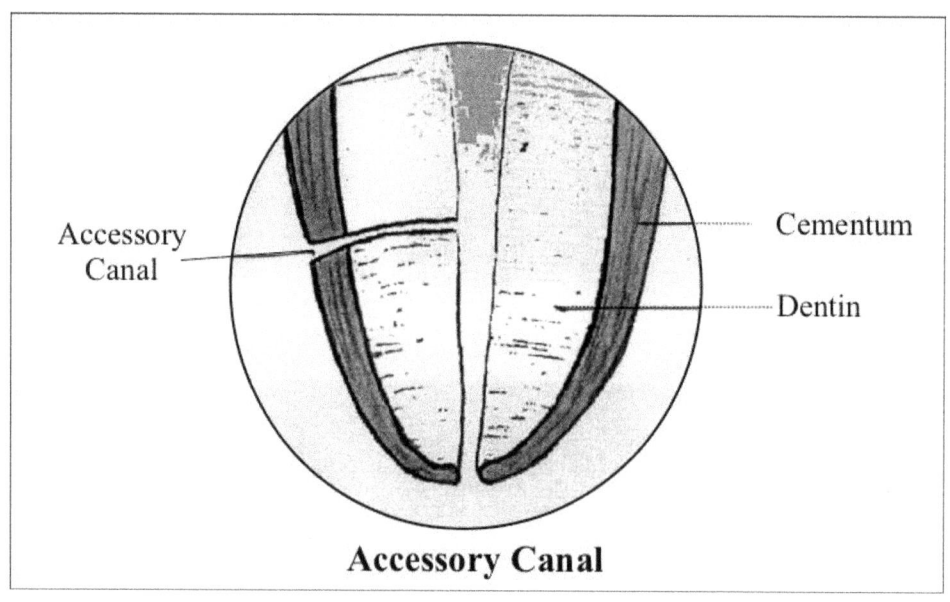

Accessory Canal

****

Q3) Functions of pulp.

Answer -- The dental pulp is the soft, highly vascularized and innervated connective tissue that supports dentin. Pulp executes the subsequent functions......

- *Inductive* – Initially the pulp, referred to as dental papilla, collaborates with the oral epithelial cells, resulting in the development of an enamel organ. It also engages with the forming enamel organ to specify a certain form of tooth.
- *Formative*– Odontoblasts are the cells that are derived from dental papilla (primitive dental pulp). These cells secrete the organic matrix of dentin and contribute to its mineralization.
- *Nutritive* – Provides nourishment to dentin through odontoblasts and their extensions, as well as through the rich vascular system present in the pulp.
- *Protective*– The pulp's sensory nerves respond to a variety of stimuli, such as heat and cold, with pain.
- *Defensive/reparative*– The pulp reacts to stimulation by generating reparative dentin. It occludes the damaged dentinal tubules through mineralization, therefore protecting the pulp from irritation. The defense cells in the pulp such as lymphocytes and neutrophils, will facilitate the repair of damaged pulp. The formation of reparative dentin and sclerotic dentin is regarded as the pulp's effort to isolate itself from irritants.

****

Q4) Odontoblasts.

Answer–

▸ The production of the dentin matrix and subsequent calcification are carried out by odontoblasts, the second most common cell type in the pulp.

▸ They are situated next to the pre-dentin or inside the odontoblastic zone of the pulp, with their cell bodies located in pulp and their extensions/processes extending into the dentinal tubules.

▸ Compared to the root region, the crown has bigger odontoblasts.

▸ The number of dentinal tubules is equal to the number of odontoblasts.

▸ Shape and organelle content of odontoblasts vary depending on their functional activity. Active cells possess elongated columnar body and prominent oval nuclei located in the basal region of the cell. Abundant rER, golgi apparatus and many mitochondria are located next to the nucleus. Inactive cells are small, possessing minimal cytoplasm and a reduced quantity of organelles.

▸ Odontoblasts have a tall columnar body in crown, a cuboidal form in the mid-root region, and an ovoid to spindle shape at the root apex. They are in close proximity to one another and are connected by junctional complexes.

▸ Adjacent to the pulp-predentin junction, the cellular cytoplasm lacks organelles. Here the cell constricts and forms a cell process that enters the dentinal tubule as odontoblastic process.

▸ The life span of odontoblasts corresponds to that of a functional tooth. They are terminal cells as they cannot undergo further division. After death, they are substituted by the differentiation of cells from the cell-rich zone in pulp.

****

Q5) Regressive changes in pulp

Q) Age changes in the pulp.

Answer –*The following changes take place in pulp with ageing……*

Cellular changes

▸ Cells in the pulp are reduced in number and size. Their cytoplasmic organelles are also reduced and their process becomes thin and short.

▸ Fibroblasts are also reduced in number and size. They show less cytoplasm and thin, long cytoplasmic processes. Mitochondria and endoplasmic reticulum numbers are also decreased.

▸ The quantity of undifferentiated ectomesenchymal cells diminishes with advancing age. This decrease in number diminishes the regeneration ability of the pulp.

Fibrosis

- Older pulps show generalized increase in collagen fiber bundles.
- Fibers are arranged longitudinally in radicular pulp and haphazardly in coronal pulp.
- An increase in collagen fibers is also seen around the blood vessels.

Pulp stones

- Refer to short notes Q1 in chapter 'Pulp'.

Vascular changes

- Blood flow diminishes because of a reduction in the quantity of blood vessels.
- Atherosclerotic plaques may form in the pulp blood vessels.
- Ultrastructural changes also appear in the basement membrane and endothelial cells of blood vessels.

***

Q6) Calcifications in the pulp / Pulp calcifications.

Answer— Refer to short notes Q1 in chapter 'Pulp'.

***

Q7) Undifferentiated mesenchymal cells.

Answer –

- Undifferentiated mesenchymal cells constitute the predominant cell type in immature pulp.
- Only a few numbers are observed following the completion of the root.
- They are larger than fibroblasts and exhibit a polyhedral morphology. They exhibit a spindle shape from the lateral view, characterized by processes and prominent oval nuclei.
- They are located in the cell-rich zone and pulp core in addition to the blood vessels.
- Their number decreases in old age. Due to this, the regenerative capacity of the pulp is decreased.

Function -- They are believed to be multipotent cells which depending upon the stimulus can transform either into odontoblasts, fibroblasts or macrophages when the need arises.

***

Q8) Clinical considerations of pulp

Answer – For endodontic and restorative treatments, understanding the dimensions and morphology of the pulp chamber and its extension into the cusp, referred to as the pulp horn, is essential.

- Young persons have wide pulp chambers, so deep cavity preparation should be avoided.
- As aging progresses, the pulp chamber diminishes in size due to ongoing dentin deposition on its roof and floor. This may hinder the identification of the canal orifice during root canal therapy.
- In elderly people, there are chances of formation of pulp stones. Their position near the entrance of the root canal may complicate the identification of the canals. They also create difficulty in cleaning the canals.
- If pulp is accidentally opened, its vitality can still be preserved if it is notinfected. This can be done by proper pulp capping procedure, which forms a dentin bridge at the site of exposure.
- Since dehydration causes pulpal damage, proper water spray should be used during tooth cutting and cavity preparation.
- Deep restorations may directly transmit heat and cold to the pulp. Hence appropriate cavity base and sub-base should be used for deeper restorations.
- Pulpal hyperplasia in young adult and adolescentsis characterized clinically as a mass of red granulation tissue called a "pulp polyp" that protrudes from the carious molar tooth. The tooth needs to be treated by endodontic procedure or extraction.
- Understanding the morphology and position of the apical foramen aids in preventing instruments from proceeding farther it during endodontic treatment.
- Pulpal inflammation may at times cause internal resorption of the tooth resulting in pink-appearing pulp tissue when seen through translucent enamel ('pink tooth'). The tooth requires endodontic therapy.

****

Q9) Nerves of dental pulp

Q) Innervation of pulp.

Answer – The pulp is well supplied with nerves. Nerves penetrate the pulp via the apical foramen along side blood vessels. They split to create a plexus in the acellular region of pulp, situated just under the odontoblastic zone on the crown of the tooth (*subodontoblastic plexus of Raschkow*). Nerve axons from this plexus traverse the cellular and acellular zones of the pulp. They either terminate near the odontoblast layer or pass with the odontoblast processes in the dentinal tubules. No such plexus exists in the root. Ascending nerves in the root, branch at regular intervals and further subdivide to supply its area. Most dental nerve bundles contain sensory afferent fibers from the fifth (trigeminal) nerve and superior ganglion sympathetic branches. There are myelinated and unmyelinated fibers. Large myelinated fibers transmit pain response. Due to the presence of only free nerve endings in the pulp, pain is the only sensation experienced, regardless of stimuli such as cold, heat, or pressure. Myelinated fibers convey intense pain, whereas unmyelinated fibers communicate dull pain.

****

Q10) Compare and contrast ameloblasts and odontoblasts.

Answer –

CONTRAST		
	Ameloblast	**Odontoblast**
1.	They synthesize enamel.	They synthesize dentin.
2.	They are originate from the cells of the IEE.	They differentiate from the cells of dental papilla.
3.	They do not have cell processes.	They have odontoblastic process that runs in the dentinal tubules.
4.	Upon the complete formation of enamel thickness, the ameloblasts stop secreting enamel matrix. It forms a stratified squamous epithelial lining (reduced enamel epithelium) that protects the newly formed enamel.	Throughout life, odontoblasts produce dentin.
5.	It differentiates after odontoblasts.	Odontoblasts initially differentiate under the influence of inner enamel epithelial cells.

COMPARE		
	Ameloblast	**Odontoblast**
1.	Generate the hard tissue of the tooth (enamel), which constitutes outermost layer of the tooth.	Produce the dentin, the tooth's hard tissue that makes up the major volume of the tooth.
2.	Tall columnar cells with numerous cytoplasmic organelles during the active period of enamel production.	Tall columnar cells with many cytoplasmic organelles during the active phase of dentinogenesis.

****

Q11) Compare and contrast radicular pulp and coronal pulp.

Answer –

	CONTRAST	
	Coronal pulp	**Radicular pulp**
1.	It is located centrally within the crown portion of the tooth	It is situated in the root section of the tooth.
2.	A tooth has single coronal pulp.	Its number may vary depending on the number of roots.
3.	Odontoblasts are tall columnar.	Odontoblasts are cuboidal to spindle-shaped.
4.	Cell-free zone of Weil is prominent.	This zone is usually absent.
5.	Cell-rich zone is prominent.	Cell-rich zone is less prominent.
6.	Collagen fibers are arranged haphazardly	Collagen fibers are arranged longitudinally.
7.	Linear calcification is uncommon.	It is more common.
8.	Pulp stones are common.	Pulp stones are rare.
9.	Subodontoblastic plexus of Raschkow is present.	This nerve plexus is absent.
10.	Pulp horn is present.	Pulp horn is absent.

	COMPARE	
	Coronal pulp	**Radicular pulp**
1.	All four zones exist in both coronal and radicular pulp.	
2.	Both are richly innervated.	
3.	Size reduces with ageing due to continuous deposition of dentin.	
4.	Calcification is common in aged pulp.	

****

Q12) Odontogenic zone / region of pulp.

Answer--

- Odontogenic zone is the outermost zone of pulp.
- It consists of odontoblasts that create a layer at the boundary of the pulp. It is the second most prevalent cell type in the pulp.
- Refer short notes Q4 in chapter 'Pulp'.

****

CEMENTUM

SHORT NOTES

Q1) Types of cementum.

Answer -- *Cementum is a dense, avascular connective tissue that protects the root or roots of teeth.*

- Cementum can be categorized into many types based on location, structure, function, formation rate, content and mineralization degree.

Based on Presence or absence of cells

- Cellular cementum
- Acellular cementum

Based on the presence or absence of fibers

- Fibrillar cementum
- Afibrillar cementum

Based onthenature and origin of collagen fibers of the matrix

- Acellular extrinsic fiber cementum
- Acellular intrinsic fiber cementum
- Acellular Afibrillar cementum
- Acellular mixed fiber cementum
- Cellular intrinsic fiber cementum
- Cellular mixed fiber cementum
- Cellular mixed stratified cementum

****

Q2) Functions of cementum.

Answer – *Cementum performs the following functions……*

Anchorage

- Cementum acts as a platform for the attachment of main fibers of the PDL, thus securing the tooth firmly within the alveolar bone socket.
- Hypophosphatasia is a condition where there is complete absence of cementum. In such cases, due to the absence of cementum, there is a lack of attachment of the periodontal ligament fibers. This consequently results in loosening and premature loss of teeth.

- As the cementum's superficial layer ages, a new layer is formed. The development of a new cementum layer maintains the attachment and secures the tooth firmly within the socket.

Adaptation

- Cementum plays role in the functional adaptation of teeth. For ex., occlusal wear leads to loss of contact between opposing teeth. After occlusal wear, opposing tooth contact is maintained by deposition of cementum in the apical region of the root.

Repair

- Damage caused to the roots due to resorption, fracture,etc, is repaired by the deposition of new cementum.

****

Q3) Hyaline layer of Hopewell smith.

Q) Intermediate cementum.

Answer –It is also referred to as intermediate cementum / hyaline layer of Hopewell smith.

- It is an unstructured layer located between the Tome's granular layer in dentin and secondary cementum.
- This layer does not exhibit features of either cementum or dentin.
- It is more mineralized than the adjacent dentin or the cementum.
- *Site* -- It is rarely seen in incisors and primary teeth, but it is seen in the apical two-thirds of molar and premolar roots.
- It may be seen throughout the length of the root or may be found in isolated areas.
- Its function although not clear, is thought to seal the sensitive root dentin.

****

Q4) Sharpey's fibers.

Answer-- On one side, the cementum and on the other, the alveolar bone, anchor the collagen fiber bundles of PDL. The embedded segment of collagen fiber bundles within the bone and cementum is known as Sharpey's fibers (SF).

- SF at the cementum is abundant although smaller in size than those at the alveolar bone.
- SF in the cementum and bone undergo partial mineralization. Mineralization takes place perpendicular to the longitudinal axis of the collagen fibers. On the alveolar bone's surface, the mineralized Sharpey's fibers appear as tiny projections.
- The primary acellular cementum contains fully mineralized Sharpey's fibers. Whereas the cellular cementum and bone shows incomplete mineralizationon the outer surface.

- A limited number of SF traverses the interdental bone of the alveolar process without interruption (*transalveolar fibers*). They may persist as the principal fibers of the neighboring periodontal ligament or intermix with the periosteum's fibers that envelope the cortical plates buccally and lingually.

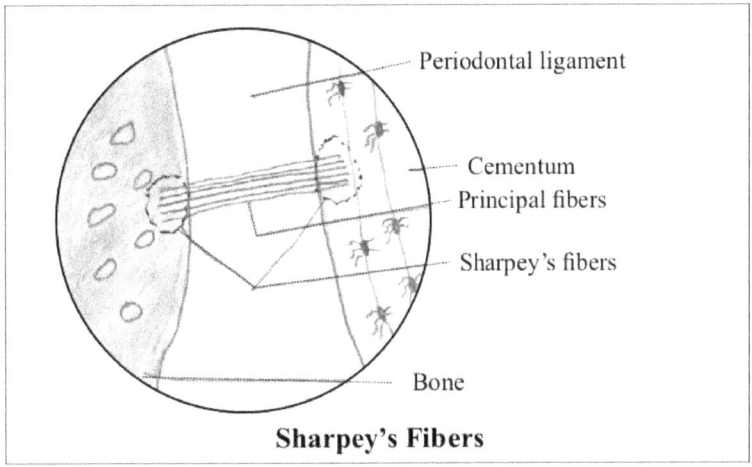

Sharpey's Fibers

****

Q5) Differences between cellular and acellular cementum.

Answer --

	Acellular cementum	**Cellular cementum**
1	Cementocytes are absent	Cementocytes are present
2	It is formed first.	This is formed after acellular cementum.
3	Also called as primary cementum.	Also called secondary cementum.
4	*Width* -- constant.	*Width* – variable.
5	*Site* – cervical area of tooth.	*Site* – Apical third and interradicular region of the root. A thin coating typically covers every root.
6	*Rate of formation* -- is slow	*The rate of formation* -- is faster.
7	*Incremental lines* – Regular and placed closely.	*Incremental lines* – irregular and widely placed.
8	Sharpey's fibers are well mineralized.	They are partially mineralized.

****

Q6) Incremental lines of Salter.

Answer-- Incremental lines in cementum are referred to as the *incremental lines of Salter*.

- They are best seen in decalcified sections.
- They represent periodic formation of cementum.
- Cellular and acellular cementum are parted apart by incremental lines. As acellular cementum is formed slowly, these lines are regular and closer. In cellular cementum, it is irregular and widely placed as this is formed at a faster rate.
- Incremental lines of Salter are characterized by significant mineralization, reduced collagen content and increased ground material compared to adjacent places.

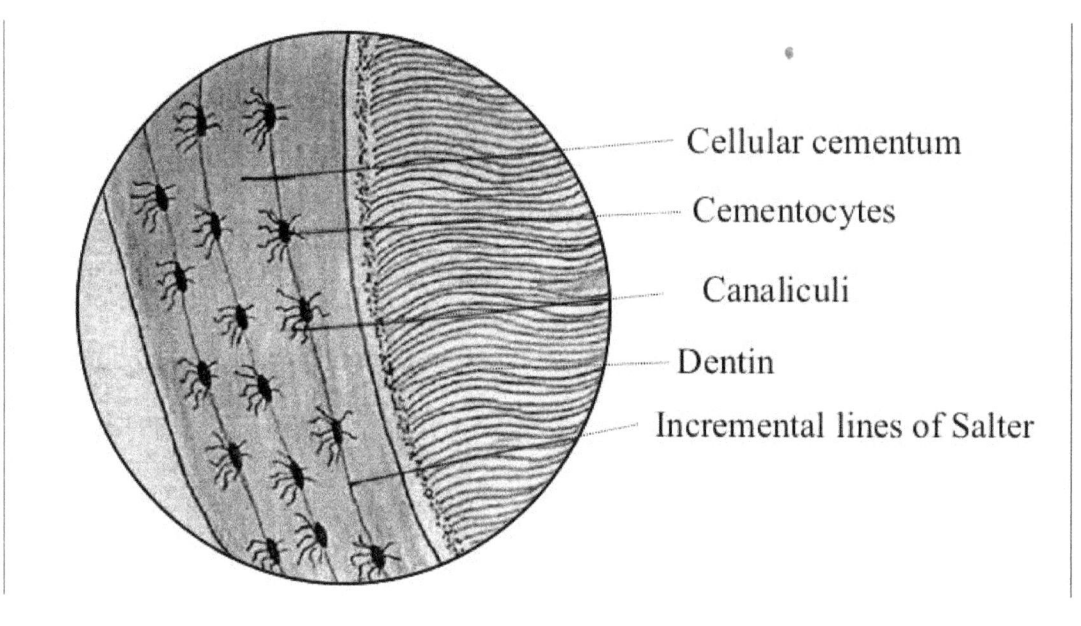

****

Q7) Cementoenamel junction (CEJ).

Answer -- The junction between cementum and enamel is called as *cementoenamel junction (CEJ)*. The scanning electron microscopic examination of the ground section reveals different types of this junction.

There are three types of cementoenamel junctions…..

1] *Cementum overlapping enamel* -- Cementum covers the enamel for a brief distance in 60% of teeth. The reduced enamel epithelium safe guards the freshly produced enamel. When it degenerates prematurely in the cervical area, the adjacent connective tissue directly contacts the enamel. Cells within the connective tissue differentiate into cementoblasts. These cells are responsible for the deposition of cementum over enamel.

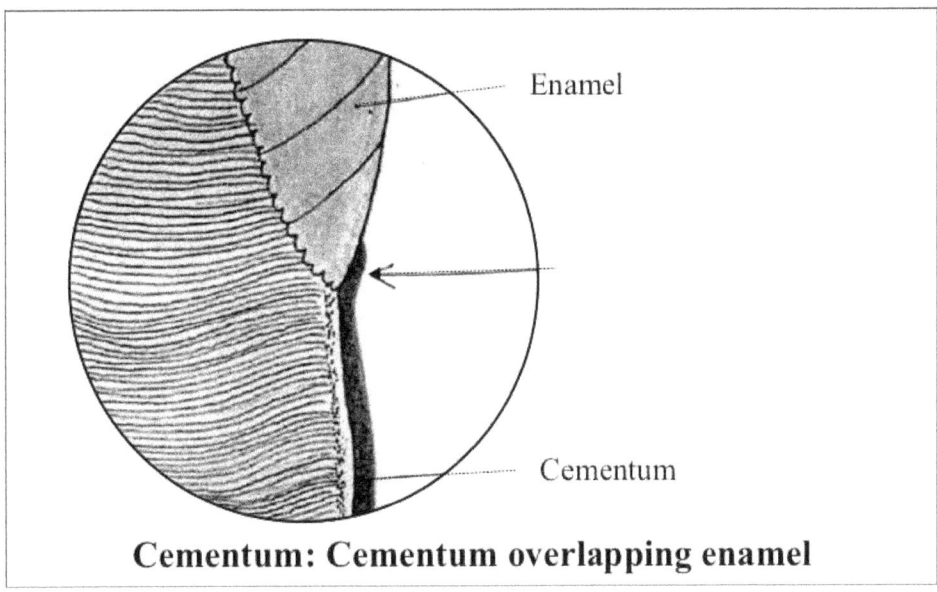
Cementum: Cementum overlapping enamel

2] *Cementum just meeting enamel (sharp junction)*--In 30% of teeth, cementum contacts with enamel at a distinct line.

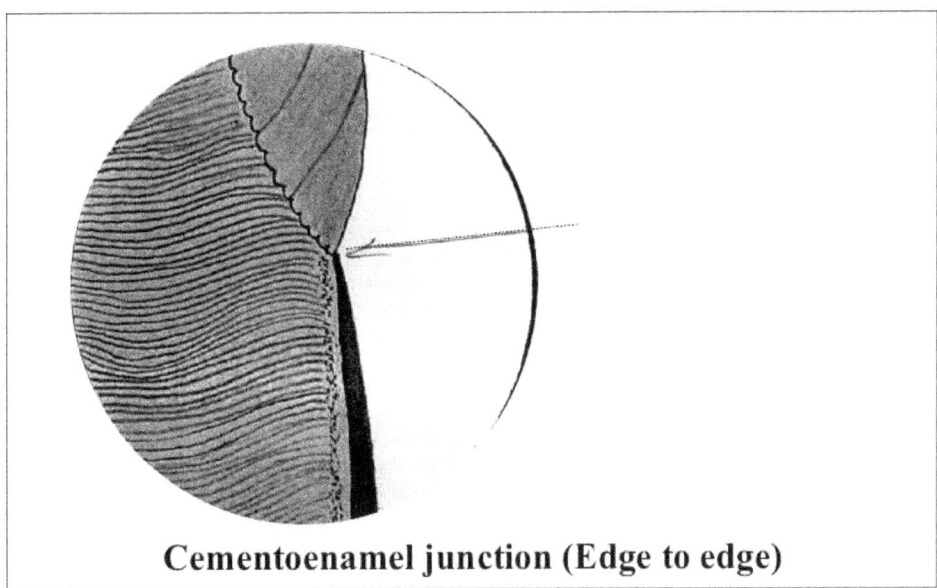
Cementoenamel junction (Edge to edge)

3] *Gap junction* -- In 10% of teeth, the cementum and enamel do not converge. A minor gap exists between them and there is an absence of a cementoenamel connection. This could occur due to a delay in the separation of reduced enamel epithelium at the cervical region of the root. The root in this area which lacks cementum may be temporarily covered by REE. Exposed root dentin at the cervical region might result in tooth sensitivity, root caries, and root resorption.

- In primary teeth, sharp junction is common, followed by cementum overlapping enamel. Gap type junction is rare in deciduous teeth.

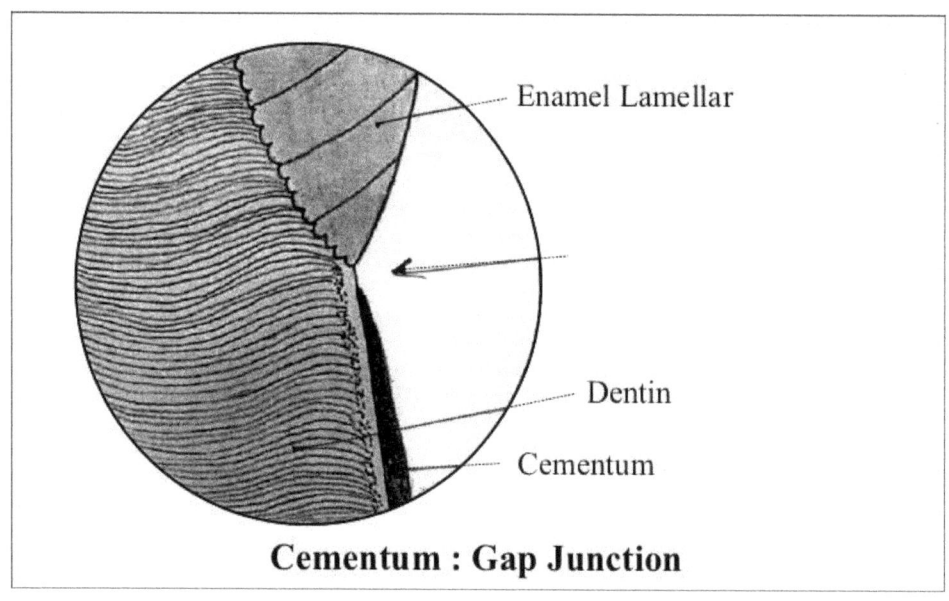

Cementum : Gap Junction

****

Q8) Cementicles.

Answer -- Cementicles are calcified, ovoid, or spherical nodules located within the periodontal ligament. They may be single cementicle or many and are situated adjacent to the cemental surface.

Cause – Aging, trauma.

Origin – The exact origin remains unclear. Degenerated HERS cells within the PDL may serve as a source for calcification.

Types

- *Free cementicles* – These cementicles are lying freely in the periodontal ligament.
- *Attached cementicles* – These Cementicles are partly fused or attached with the cementum surface.
- *Embedded cementicles* – These cementicles are completely enclosed within the cementum. Initially, they will be lying freely in the ligament. But with continued cementumdeposition,initially these get attached to it (attached cementicles) and later get embedded in the cementum.

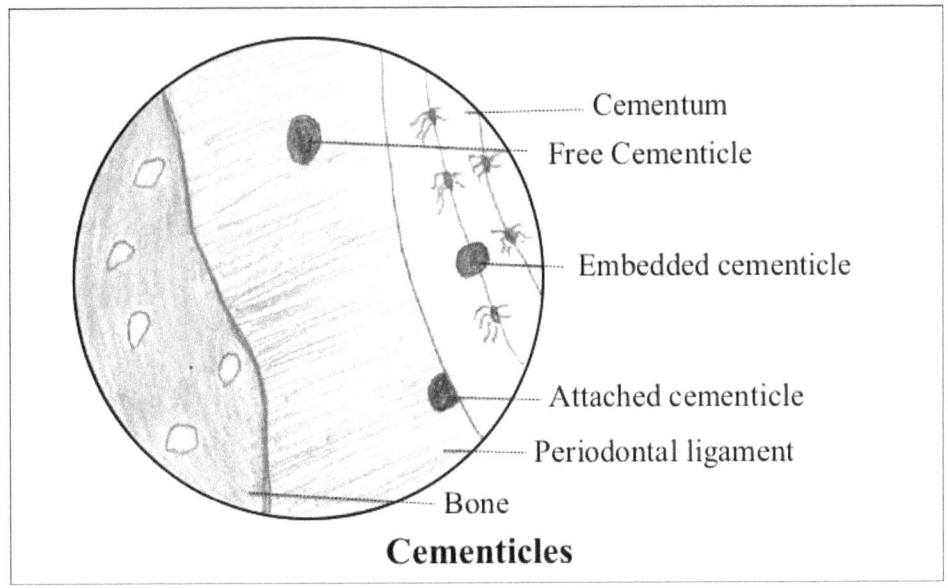

Cementicles

****

Q9) Cementogenesis.

Answer --Formation of cementum is called cementogenesis.

- The cementum is formed along the root's entire surface.
- HERS is a cervical extension of IEE and OEE. It sends inductive signal totheectomesenchymalcells in the dental papilla. These peripheral ectomesenchymal cells will now differentiate into odontoblasts (dentin-forming cells) and start secreting root predentin along the inner aspect of the root sheath. After dentin deposition, the odontoblasts retract inwards without leaving their process.
- Once the dentin formation starts, break occurs in the Hertwig'sepithelial root sheath thereby allowing the newly formed dentin to come in direct contact with the connective cells of the dental follicle. The inner cells of the dental follicle differentiate into cementoblasts. Cementoblasts are the cells that synthesize collagen and protein polysaccharides which make up the organic matrix of the cementum.
- After some cementum matrix has been laid down, its mineralization begins. The uncalcified matrix is called *cementoid.* It gets mineralized by addition of calcium and phosphorous ions present in tissue fluids.
- Formation of cementum is a rhythmic process. As a new layer of cementoid is formed, the old one calcifies. A thin layer of cementoid lined by cementoblasts is seen on the outer cemental surface.
- Collagen fibers from the adjacent periodontal ligament pass in between the cementoblasts and are embedded into the cementum. These fibers firmly anchor the tooth to the surrounding bone. These embedded portions of the fibers are known as *Sharpey's fibers.*

****

Q10) Hypercementosis.

Answer -- Hypercementosis is a term used to describe abnormal thickening of cementum.

- This occurs in teeth that are subjected to high stress.
- Hypercementosis can be either diffuse (involving the entire root surface) or may be circumscribed (localized to a particular part of the root and more commonly the apex).
- It may impact every tooth or affect an individual tooth.
- If the cemental overgrowth improves the cementum's functional properties, it is known as *cementum hypertrophy*.
- *Cementum hyperplasia* is defined as cemental overgrowth occurring in nonfunctional teeth or when it fails to enhance functional quality.
- Extensive cemental hyperplasia is sometimes related to chronic periapical inflammation. It appears as circumscribed mass surrounding the root as a cuff.
- Generalized hypercementosis is seen in Paget's disease and localized form in benign cemetoblastoma, fluorid cemento-osseous dysplasia, etc.

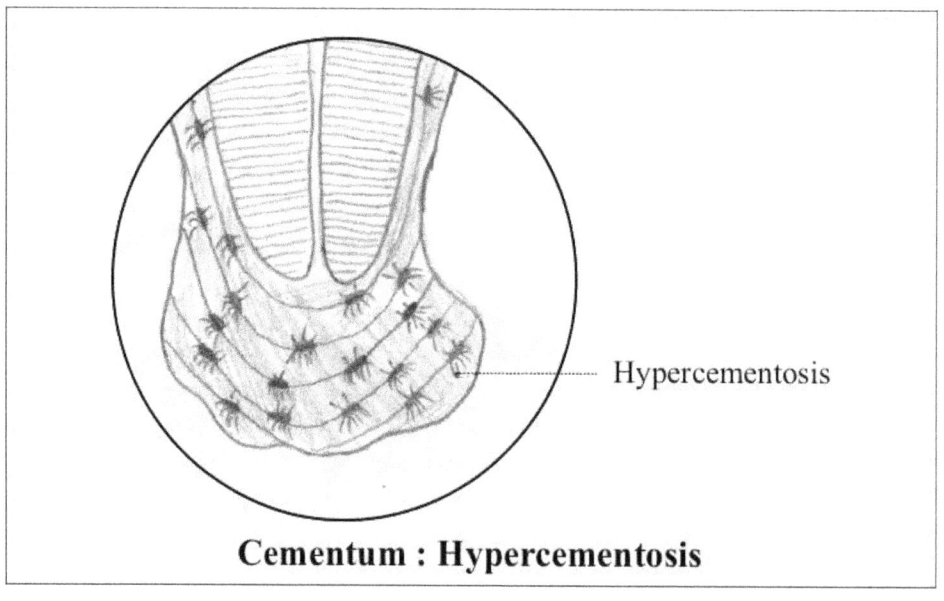

Cementum : Hypercementosis

****

Q11) Hertwig's epithelial root sheath.

Answer --

- The enamel organ is essential for the development of HERS.
- HERS shapes the root and initiates the development of root dentin.
- Upon complete formation of crown, the IEE and OEE cells at the cervical loop undergo proliferation to form a double layer of cells referred to as HERS. It comprises only IEE and OEE.

- HERS cells impact the neighboring dental papilla cells, prompting their differentiation into odontoblasts. These odontoblasts secrete the first layer of root dentin. Once dentin is deposited, HERS breaks down and loses its continuity.
- HERS cells degenerate. But some may still remain as remnants in the periodontal ligament as isolated islands or nests or interconnecting strands close to cemental surface. These are known as *cells rest of Malassez.*
- The premature loss of root sheath cells may result in the development of an auxiliary canal within the pulp. Dental papilla cells are unable to develop into odontoblasts, which are in charge of creating root dentin. Thus absence in that area may lead to the formation of direct lateral channel connecting the periodontal ligament and the pulp (accessory canal).

****

Q12) Cellular cementum.

Answer-- Cellular cementum is called so because it incorporates spider-like cementocytes in the lacunae.

- The incremental lines in cellular cementum are distantly spaced due to its gradual formation.
- Compared to acellular cementum, it has a lesser mineral content.

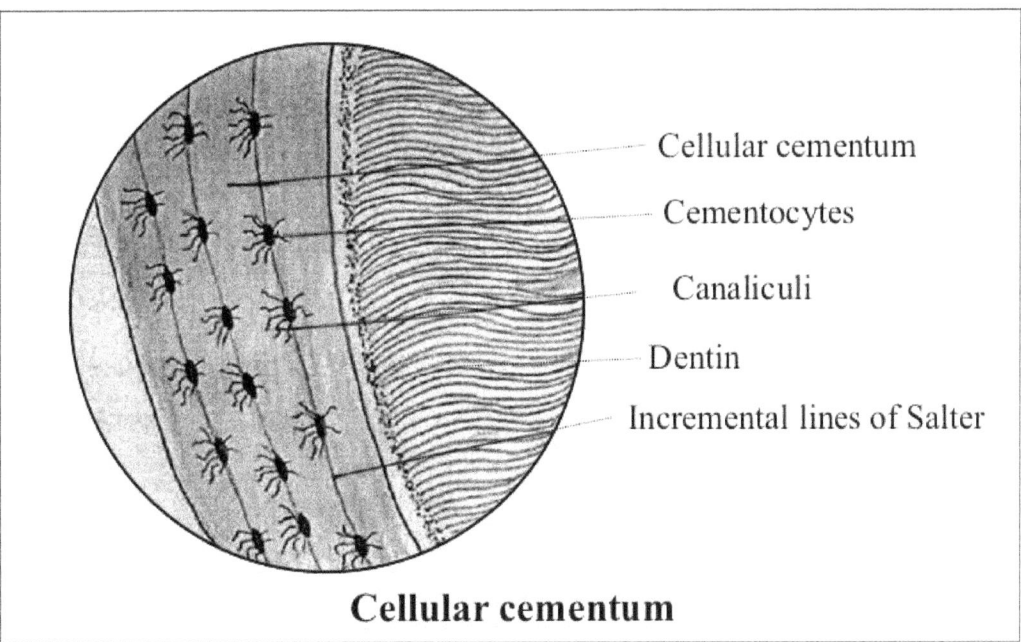

Cellular cementum

Types of cellular cementum

1) Cellular intrinsic fiber cementum
2) Cellular mixed fiber cementum.
3) Cellular mixed stratified cementum.

CELLULAR INTRINSIC FIBER CEMENTUM / SECONDARY CEMENTUM

- Cellular intrinsic fiber cementumis called so because it consists of cells (cementocytes) incorporated in it and its fibers are derived from cementoblasts (intrinsic fibers). It is also called secondary cementum, as it forms later in life i.e. after the tooth comes in occlusion.
- *Cementocytes* – during cementum deposition, the cementoblasts that release the cementum's organic matrix become caught in it. The cementoblasts that become imprisoned are referred to as cementocytes. They inhabit spaces known as lacunae and possess several processes or canaliculi extending from their bodies toward the periodontal ligament, which serves as their nutritional source. Their canaliculi may diverge and converge with those of adjacent cementocytes, thus preserving communication. Cementocytes in the deep layers are less active and contain only few organelles indicating that they are degenerating. Cementocytes in much deeper layers show definite signs of degeneration. Further deeper in the cementum, only empty lacunae are visible which suggests complete degeneration of cementocytes. Most cementocytes are seen in the apical third of the root.
- *Intrinsic fibers* -- Cementoblasts generate fine, parallel-to-the-root surface intrinsic fibers. The cellular intrinsic fiber cementum does not help in tooth anchorage due to lack of extrinsic fibers from PDL.
- *Location*– Middle third to apical third of the root and interradicular areas.
- *Functions*– Adaptation, repair.

CELLULAR MIXED FIBER CEMENTUM

- It is called so because it consists of cells (cementocytes) incorporated in it and its fibers are derived from both cementoblasts (intrinsic fibers) and fibroblasts of the periodontal ligament (extrinsic fibers).
- As it is formed rapidly, it is less mineralized.
- It forms the main bulk of secondary cementum.
- *Cementocytes* – As cementum is deposited, the cementoblasts that secrete the organic matrix of cementum become caught within the matrix they produce. The cementoblasts that become embraced within the cemental matrix are referred to as cementocytes. They inhabit spaces known as lacunae and possess several processes or canaliculi extending from their bodies towards the periodontal ligament, which serves as their nutritional source. Their processes may branch and join with those of adjacent cementocytes, hence maintaining the communication. Cementocytes in the deep layers are less active and contain only few organelles indicating that they are degenerating. Cementocytes in much deeper layers show definite signs of degeneration. Further deeper in the cementum, only empty lacunae are visible which suggests complete degeneration of cementocytes. Most cementocytes are seen in the apical third of the root.
- *Intrinsic and extrinsic fibers* – Cementoblasts produce the intrinsic fibers which are finer and smaller than the extrinsic fibers. They run parallel to the surface of the roots. Fibroblasts in the PDL produce extrinsic fibers that are directed perpendicular to the root surface.

- *Location* -- Apical third and furcation areas of the root.
- *Function* – Adaptation.

CELLULAR MIXED STRATIFIED CEMENTUM

- Cellular mixed stratified cementum gets its name from the alternating layers of cellular intrinsic fiber cementum and acellular extrinsic fiber cementum.
- *Cementocytes* –As cementum is deposited, the cementoblasts that secrete the organic matrix of cementum become caught within the matrix they produce. The cementoblasts that become imprisoned are referred to as cementocytes. They inhabit spaces known as lacunae and possess several processes or canaliculi extending from their bodies toward the periodontal ligament, which serves as their nutritional source. Their process may branch and joins with those of adjacent cementocytes, preserving communication. Cementocytes in the deep layers are less active and contain only few organelles indicating that they are degenerating. Cementocytes in much deeper layers show definite signs of degeneration. Further deeper in the cementum, only empty lacunae are visible which suggests complete degeneration of cementocytes. Most cementocytes are seen in the apical third of the root.
- *Intrinsic and extrinsic fibers* –The intrinsic fibers produced by cementoblasts are finer and smaller than the extrinsic fibers. They run parallel to the root surface. Perpendicular to the root surface is extrinsic fibers produced by fibroblasts in the periodontal ligament.
- *Site* – Apical third and furcation areas of the root.

****

Q13) Acellular cementum.

Answer -- Acellular cementum is called so because of the absence of cementocytes in it.

Types of acellular cementum

1) Acellular intrinsic fiber cementum.

2) Acellular extrinsic fiber cementum / Primary cementum.

3) Acellular afibrillar cementum.

4) Acellular mixed fiber cementum.

ACELLULAR INTRINSIC FIBER CEMENTUM

- It is the first formed cementum.
- It is acellular (i.e. does not contain cementocytes) and its fibers are derived from cementoblasts.

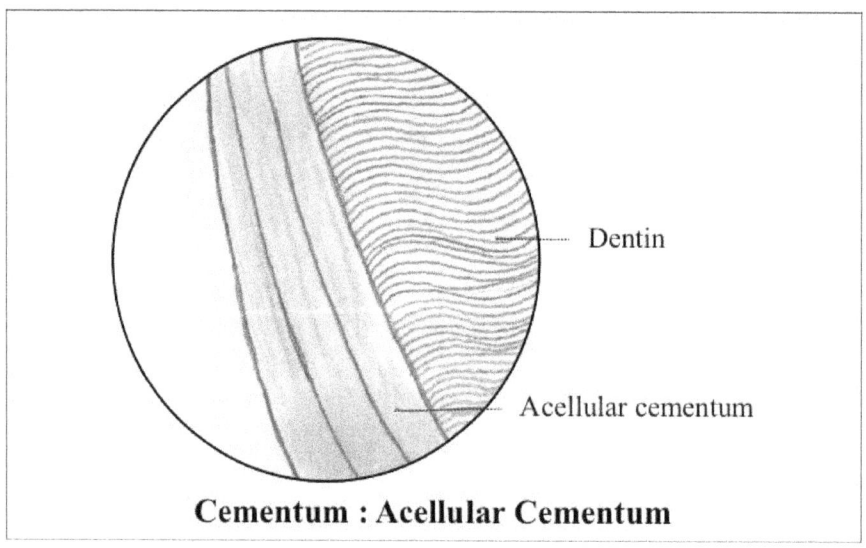

Cementum : Acellular Cementum

ACELLULAR EXTRINSIC FIBER CEMENTUM / PRIMARY CEMENTUM

- It is usually considered as primary cementum as it formed first.
- It is acellular (i.e. does not contain cementocytes) and its fibers are derived from fibroblasts in the periodontal ligament.
- It surrounds two-thirds of the root and constitutes major volume of the root.
- The incremental lines are closely spaced and parallel, due to its gradual and regular formation.
- The acellular extrinsic fiber cementum's innermost layer exhibits less mineralization. The outer layer shows alternative more mineralized and less mineralized areas parallel to the root surface.
- *Extrinsic fibers* -- The extrinsic fibers are secreted by fibroblasts of the PDL. They are known as Sharpey's fibers and pierce the cementum at a right angle to the surface. These fibers are predominantly mineralized, with the exception of their core, which remains unmineralized.
- *Location*–from the root's apical third to cervical boundary.
- *Function*-- Anchoring the tooth to the socket.

ACELLULAR AFIBRILLAR CEMENTUM

- This cementum is acellular (i.e. does not contain cementocytes) and does not contain both intrinsic and extrinsic fibers.
- It is observed as a fine coating over both the dentin and enamel surface, adjacent to the cementoenamel junction.
- Due to absence of intrinsic and extrinsic fibers, it has no role to play in tooth attachment.
- The cells laying this cementum remain unidentified. Previously, it was considered a developmental abnormality resulting from the premature loss of the reduced enamel epithelium that protects the newly produced enamel. The dental follicle cells will now contact the freshly created enamel, develop into cementoblasts, and synthesize this cementum.

****

Q14) Cementoblasts.

Answer -- Cementoblasts are the cells that form cementum. They line the surface of both cellular and acellular cementum. They synthesize collagen and proteins that constitute the organic matrix of cementum. These active cells possess numerous organelles involved in synthesis and secretion, including the golgi apparatus, rough endoplasmic reticulum, and mitochondria.

- Adjacent cementoblasts are attached by junctional complexes.
- As cementum matrix is deposited, the cementoblasts that secrete it become caught within the same matrix. The cementoblasts that become confined within the cemental matrix are referred to as *cementocytes*.
- *Differentiation/ Formation*– HERS transmit inductive signals to neighboring dental papilla cells prompting their differentiation into odontoblasts. The odontoblasts produce the root dentin's first layer. Upon the formation of root dentin, the HERS disintegrates and its previous continuity is lost. This will allow the inner cells of dental follicle to contact the freshly created dentin. The inner cells develop into cementoblasts.

****

Q15) Cementocytes.

Answer – As cementum is deposited, the cementoblasts that secrete the organic matrix of cementum become caught within the matrix they produce. The cementoblasts that become embraced within the cemental matrix are referred to as cementocytes.

- They are present in compartments known as lacunae and possess several processes or canaliculi extending from their bodies towards the periodontal ligament, which serves as their nutritional source. Their processes branch and join with the processes of neighboring cementocytes, thus maintaining their communication.
- Cementocytes in the deep layers are less active and contain only few organelles indicating that they are degenerating.
- Cementocytes in much deeper layers show definite signs of degeneration. Further deeper in the cementum, only empty lacunae are visible which suggests complete degeneration of cementocytes.
- They are similar to osteocytes in bone, but their lacunae are ovoid/tubular, unlike osteocyte lacunae which are oval. They have fewer canaliculi than osteocytes.
- The majority of cementocytes are located in the apical part of the root.

****

Q16) Cementodentinal junction (CDJ).

Answer – The junction between cementum and dentin is called cementodentinal junction (CDJ). This junction is firm and is clearly visible under light microscope

- The attachment is firm. Under an electron microscope, the CDJ is a broad region that comprises a substantial amount of collagen fibers which aids in the firm binding between cementum and dentin.
- It is scalloped in primary teeth and smooth in permanent teeth.
- Cementum may sometimes be separated from dentin by a thin strip known as *intermediate cementum*. This layer characteristics of both cementum and dentin.
- The collagen fibers from both cementum and dentin intermingle at the CDJ. It is often difficult to ascertain whether the fibers are from dentin or cementum. These fibers are more in cellular cementum.

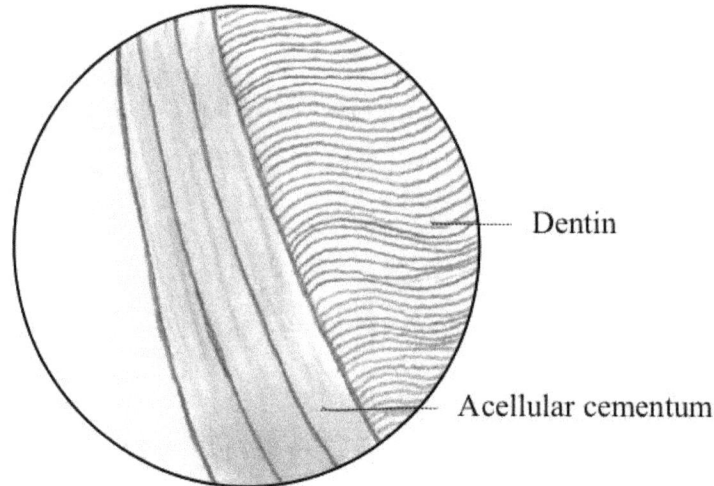

****

PERIODONTAL LIGAMENT

MAIN QUESTIONS

Q1) Define periodontium. Describe in detail the principal fibers of periodontal ligament.

Answer -- The periodontium is a connective tissue that consists of PDL, cementum, alveolar bone, and gingiva.

- The PDL is a type of soft connective tissue that is found in the periodontal space between the alveolar bone, which makes up the socket wall and the cementum of the tooth root.

PRINCIPAL FIBERS OF PERIODONTAL LIGAMENT

- The principal fibers of the PDL predominantly consist of collagen fibers organized into bundles. The bundles connecting the tooth root to the socket wall's bone are organized into various groups known as the principal fibers of PDL.
- *There are five groups of principal fibers in periodontal ligament*

    i] Alveolar crest group
    ii] Horizontal group
    iii] Oblique group
    iv] Apical group
    v] Interradicular group

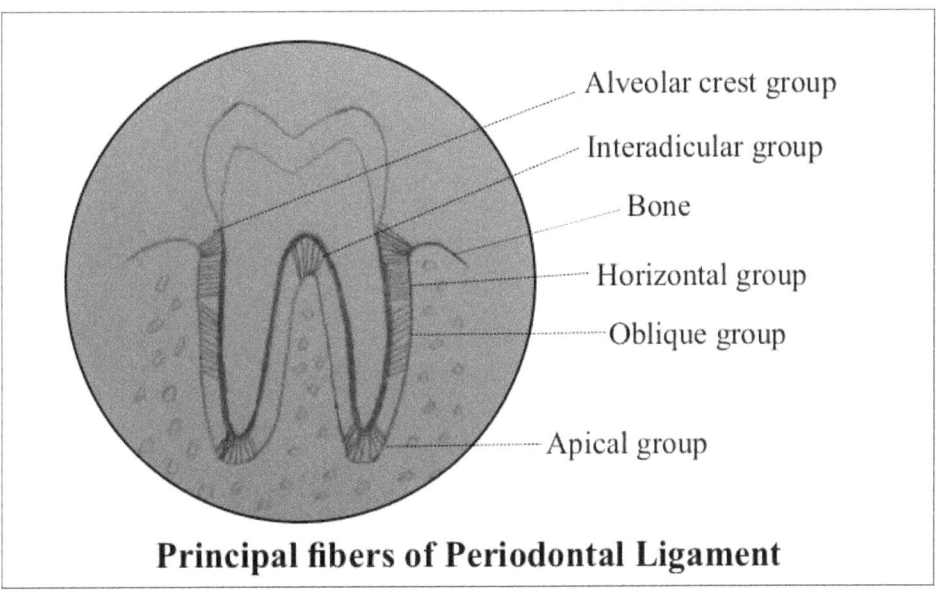

Principal fibers of Periodontal Ligament

Alveolar crest group

- Alveolar crest group fibers extend obliquely downward from the cervical cementum below the CEJ and insert into the crest of alveolar bone below.
- Certain fibers run from the alveolar crest to get inserted into the periosteum that covers the alveolar bone.

Functions

- It withstands tilting, intrusive, extrusive, and rotating pressures.

Horizontal group

- Horizontal group fibers are present just below the alveolar crest group.
- These fibers are oriented perpendicular to the long axis of the tooth. One end of this group is fixed in the alveolar bone and the other end into the cementum. *Sharpey'sfibers* is a term used for these fibers that are embedded in bone and cementum.

Functions

- It resists horizontal and tipping forces.

Oblique group

- The oblique group of fibers comprises the largest of the five groups in the periodontal ligament.
- They run obliquely from cementum belowand are inserted in bone coronally.

Functions

- This fiber group resists vertical and intrusive forces.

Apical group

This group of fibers extends from the cementum at the root apex and inserts into the bone at the base of the bony socket.

- This fiber group is not seen in incompletely formed roots.

Functions

- It resists forces of luxation and prevents tipping. It protects fragile blood vessels, nerves, and lymphatic vessels traversing from the PDL to the apical foramen.

Interradicular group

- Interradicular group fibers are observed only in multirooted teeth.
- The fibers run from cementum at the root furcation and get inserted into crest of interradicular bone.

Functions

- The fibers resist tipping forces, torquing, and luxation.

GINGIVAL FIBER GROUP

- *Gingival group of fibers (also called as gingival ligament), is also considered to be a part of the principal fibers. These fibers are located in the lamina propria (LP) of the gingiva. They provide support to free gingiva, firmly connect the attached gingiva to the alveolar bone and teeth and also connect adjacent teeth. There are five categories of gingival fibers. ....*
- Dentogingival group
- Alveologingival group
- Circular group
- Dentoperiosteal group
- Transeptal group

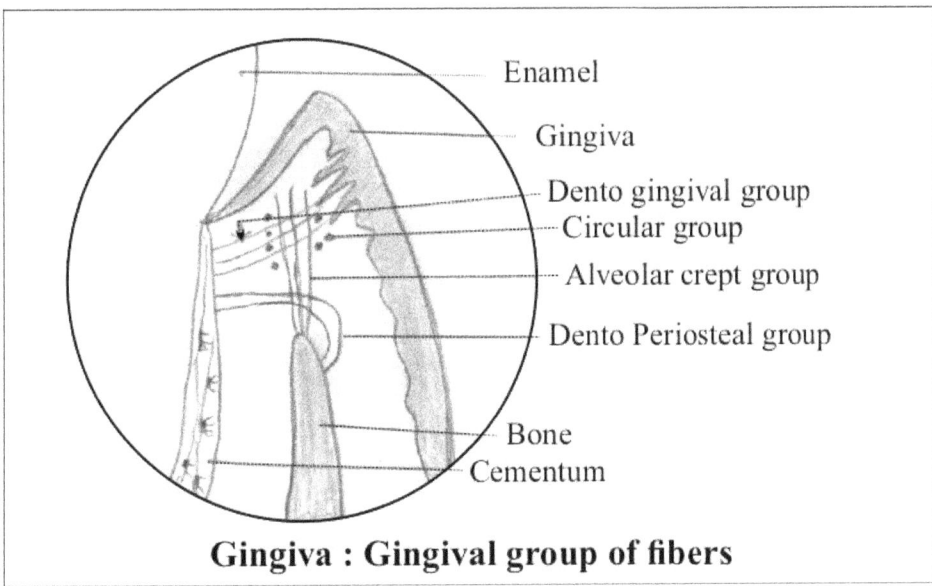

Gingiva : Gingival group of fibers

Dentogingival group

- The gingival fibers of this category is the most abundant among the five groups.
- The fibers run from the cervical cementum beneath the CEJ and are inserted in the LP of both free and attached gingiva.

Alveologingival group

- These fibers run from the crest of alveolar bone and are anchored in the LP of both the free and attached gingiva.

Circular group

- These are a small group of fibers.
- These fibers run in a circular fashion around the neck of tooth.
- This group binds the free gingiva to the tooth.

Dentoperiosteal group

- The fibers in this group run from the cervical cementum just beneath the cementoenamel junction and are anchored in the periosteum that envelops the alveolar bone's outer cortical plate.

Transeptal group

- Transeptal fibers run interdentally between two teeth. They extend from the cervical cementum beneath the CEJ of one tooth, traverse over the crest of the alveolar bone, and insert into the cementum beneath the CEJ of the adjacent tooth.

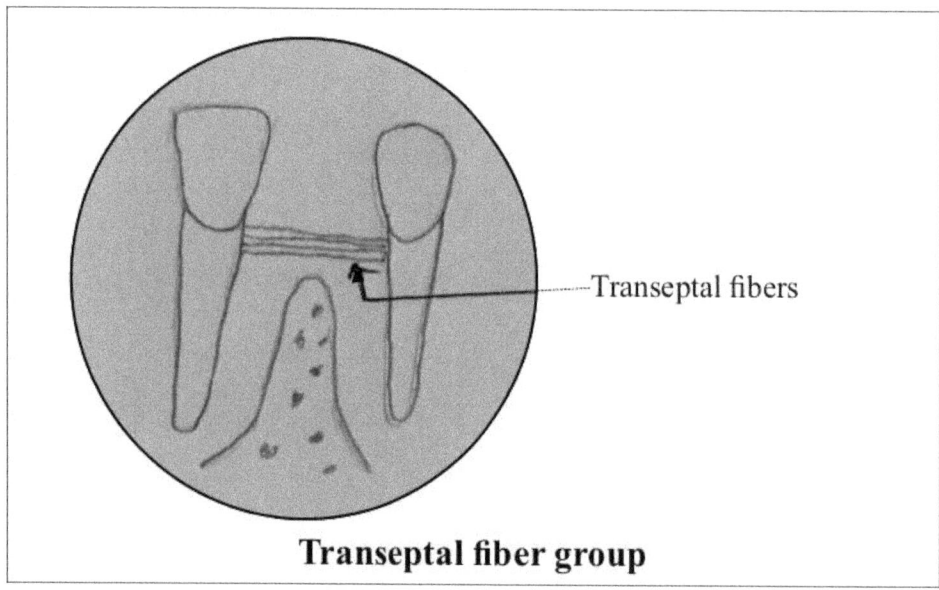

Transeptal fiber group

****

Q2) Discuss the histology of periodontal ligament with suitable diagrams.

Answer-- The PDL is a specialized soft connective tissue located in the periodontal space, present between the cementum of tooth root and the alveolar bone that constitutes the socket wall.

- Refer to section 'Cells of periodontal ligament' in short notes Q5 in chapter 'Periodontal ligament'.
- Refer to sections 'Principal fibers of periodontal ligament' and 'Gingival group of fibers' in main question Q1 in chapter 'Periodontal ligament'.
- Refer to short notes 'Sharpey's fibers' Q4 in chapter "Cementum".

****

SHORT NOTES

Q1) Principal fibers of periodontal ligament.

Answer -- Refer to section 'Principal fibers of periodontal ligament' in main question Q1 in chapter 'Periodontal ligament'

****

Q2) Transeptal fibers.

Answer --Refer to section 'Transeptal group' in main question Q1 in chapter 'Periodontal ligament'

****

Q3) Alveolar crest fibers.

Answer --Refer to section 'Alveolar crest group' in main question Q1 in chapter 'Periodontal ligament'

****

Q4) Intermediate plexus.

Answer -- Previously, it was considered that the major fibers of PDL followed a wavy path from the root's cementum to the alveolar bone of socket wall, converging in the central region of the PDL space to form a zone known as the *intermediate plexus*.

- This region was regarded as a site of excessive metabolic activity.
- As this zone is seen only in longitudinal section and not in cross section, it was later considered to be an artifact produced during tissue processing. Recent investigations indicate that the entire PDL is metabolically active, rather than solely the central region.

****

Q5) Cells of periodontal ligament.

Answer -- *Alveolar bone, cementum, and the fibrous connective tissue of the periodontal ligament are all synthesized and resorbed by cells present in the ligament. These cells are categorized as follows:*

1) <u>SYNTHETIC CELLS</u>
   Fibroblasts
   Osteotoblasts
   Cementoblasts

2) <u>RESORPTIVE CELLS</u>
   - Fibroblasts
   - Osteoclasts
   - Cementoclasts

3) <u>DEFENSE CELLS</u>
   - Mast cells
   - Macrophages
   - Eosinophils

4) <u>EPITHELIAL CELLS</u>
   - Cell rests of Malassez

5) <u>PROGENITOR CELLS</u>

FIBROBLASTS

- Fibroblasts are the principal cells in the periodontal ligament.
- They are sizable spindle or stellate-shaped cells characterized by ample cytoplasm and multiple organelles involved in synthesis of protein and its secretion, such as rER, golgi apparatus, secretory vesicles, and mitochondria.
- They are aligned with the fiber bundles. They possess elongated, slender cytoplasmic extensions that surround these fiber bundles.
- Fibroblasts contact each other by their processes and adhere to each other by cell junctions.
- In aged pulp, they have a round or spindle shape, possess short processes and contain few organelles, and are now referred to as *fibrocytes*.
- If fibroblast function is affected, there is decreased fiber synthesis leading to the loss of tooth's supporting tissue.

Functions

- Fibroblasts have dual function. They are associated with remodeling of collagen fibers i.e. they simultaneously synthesize and degrade old collagen fibers.
- They produce glycoproteins and proteoglycans which constitute the ground substance of periodontal ligament.
- They secrete collagenase, an enzyme that breaks down collagen.

OSTEOBLASTS

- Refer to short notes Q7 in chapter 'Bone'

CEMENTOBLASTS

- Refer to short notes Q14 in chapter 'Cementum'.

OSTEOCLASTS

- Refer to short notes Q9 in chapter 'Bone'

CEMENTOCLASTS

- Cementoclasts resemble osteoclasts.
- They are large mononuclear or multinuclear giant cells located in resorption bays known as Howship's lacunae on the surface of the cementum.
- They induce the resorption of cementum under specific conditions.
- Its origin is not known.

MAST CELLS

- Mast cells are typically round or oval in shape and are frequently located adjacent to blood arteries.
- They are characterized by presence of cytoplasmic granules containing heparin and histamine.
- *Functions* -- Mast cells are associated with inflammatory reactions. They release contents from their granules into the extracellular region during antigen-antibody reaction. Histamine causes mesenchymal and endothelial cells to proliferate. Mast cells contribute to the preservation of endothelial and fibroblast cell populations.

MACROPHAGES

- Macrophages are defense cells derived from monocytes in blood and are seen in association with blood vessels.
- *Functions* -- They engulf or ingest foreign matter, dead cells and microorganisms invading PDL; they also secrete growth factors that regulate proliferation of fibroblasts and endothelial cells.

EOSINOPHILS

- They are derived from blood vessels and occassionally seen in PDL.
- *Functions* – Phagocytosis.

EPITHELIAL CELLS

- Upon the formation of root dentin, Hertwig's epithelial root undergoes disintegration. Some cells of the root sheath degenerate whereas some may remain as remnants in the periodontal ligament. They are present in the form of isolated islands, nests or interlinking strands at the cemental surface. These are referred to as the *rest of Malassez cells*.
- They are abundant in the furcation areas.
- They number is less in old age and more in young individuals.
- Function of these rest cells is not clear. They may multiply to become cysts and tumors or undergo mineralization to become cementicles.

PROGENITOR CELLS

- Progenitor cells are also called undifferentiated mesenchymal cells.
- They are an essential component of the PDL cells.
- They are located around the blood vessels.
- They possess mitotic capability and serve as the origin of new cells for the ligament. The origin of fibroblasts, osteoblasts along with cementoblasts from a singular progenitor cell or distinct progenitors for each cell type remains uncertain.

****

Q6) Synthetic cells of periodontal ligament.

Answer-- Refer section 'Synthetic cells' in short notes Q5 in chapter 'Periodontal ligament'

****

Q7) Functions of periodontal ligament

Answer -- *Functions of periodontal ligament are as follows……*

Supportive - When a tooth moves within its socket due to masticatory or orthodontic pressure, a portion of the PDL will experience compression. The displaced tooth is supported by collagen fibers and water molecules present in the periodontal ligament. Oblique fiber group will help in transferring the force exerted onto the alveolar bone.

Sensory - Periodontal ligament has an efficient proprioceptive mechanism. It can even detect very delicate force on the teeth and also any slight displacement. Consequently, it safeguards both the structures that support the tooth and lessens the risk of crown fracture resulting from high masticatory forces.

Nutritive – The blood arteries in the PDL supply essential nutrients to the cells and facilitate the removal of cellular waste. Occlusion of blood vessels (due to heavy pressure during orthodontic treatment) can result in necrosis of cells in the area supplied by the vessel due to non-availability of nutrition.

Homeostatic - PDL cells possess the capability to resorb and generate extracellular matrix components of the PDL, alveolar bone, cementum. New cells obtained from the cell division of the progenitor cells replace the dead and necrotic cells.

Eruptive – Periodontal ligament has only a limited role in tooth eruption.

****

BONE

SHORT NOTES

Q1) Incremental lines of bone.

Answer – Incremental lines in bone, known as cement lines, are characterized by hypomineralization.

- These are two types – resting lines and reversal lines.
- *Resting lines* – These lines demonstrate the incremental pattern of bone formation. It marks the period of resting during bone deposition. It appears as dark blue, smooth wavy lines in H and E stained sections.
- *Reversal lines* – These lines indicate the stoppage of osteoclast activity on the surface of the bone undergoing resorption. This line defines the boundary between old and new bone that is formed. The preosteoblasts mature into osteoblasts and deposit a thin layer of non-collagenous matrix protein on the resorbed surface. This cement line contains minimal or no collagen and exhibits a high concentration of glycoproteins and proteoglycans. In H and E staining, it appears as dark blue uneven scalloped lines.

****

Q2) Types of bone.

Answer – Bone is a living tissue that constitutes the skeletal framework of the body.

Types of bone

    a) Depending upon the shape – Long bone,

                          Short bone,

                           Flat bone,

                           Irregular bone.

    b) Depending upon the development – Endochondral bone,

                                       Intramembraneous bone.

    c) Based on the histology – Mature bone,

                             Immature bone – Compact bone

                                          Cancellous bone.

****

Q3) Alveolar bone proper

Answer –The alveolar bone proper is a slender layer of bone covering the tooth root that provides attachment for the principal fibers of the PDL. It measures 0.1 – 0.4 mm in thickness and is composed of both lamellated bone and bundle bone.

- Radiographically, the alveolar bone proper has increased radiopacity, so it is additionally known as *lamina dura*. The increased radiopacity results not from enhanced mineral content but from the existence of dense bone devoid of trabeculations.

Lamellar bone

- The lamellar bone contains the basic structural unit of bone called 'osteons' or 'haversian system'.
- Concentric layers of bone are developed around a central vascular canal, called the Haversian canal. These concentric lamellae and Haversian canal collectively constitute the Osteon or Haversian system.
- In histology sections, an osteon is a long, cylindrical structure that runs parallel to the bone's long axis. Each osteon may have up to 20 concentric lamellae. A cement line, referred to as the reversal line, demarcates the Haversian systems. This line has significant basophilia and may possess minimal or no collagen.
- Adjacent Haversian canals are joined by Volkmann canals. These canals consist of blood vessels, establishing a dense vascular network within the bone.
- Osteocytes are present in lacunae located at junctions of concentric lamellae. The canaliculi of the osteocytes radiate towards the Haversian canal. This connection mechanism will facilitate the exchange of nutrients and waste with the blood vessels present in the canal. Also adjacent osteocytes interconnect with each other by their processes.
- Interstitial lamellae fill the space between adjacent haversian systems.

Bundle bone

- Bundle bone refers to the bone in which the principal fibers of the PDL are attached.
- Called as 'bundle' because of the continuation of the principal fiber bundles into the bone as Sharpey's fibers.
- Bundle bone is distinguished by a shortage of fibrils in intercellular matrix. The fibrils are arranged perpendicularly to the Sharpey's fibers.
- The slides stained with hematoxylin and eosin exhibit a black hue to the bundle bone.
- Rest lines are seen in bundle bone.
- Inner wall of the bony socket which is formed by the alveolar bone proper has numerous holes through which blood vessels and branches of interalveolar nerves enter the PDL, and is also known as the *cribriform plate*.

Interdental septum

- The interdental septum is the bone located between adjacent teeth and interradicular bone is located between the roots of mutiroooted teeth. It is made solely of the cribriform plate. The interdental and interradicular arteries, veins, lymphatic vessels are present within this perforating plate (*Zuckerkandl* and *Hirschfeld*).

****

Q4) Howship's lacunae.

Answer – Howship's lacunae is a cavity on the bony surface, created and occupied by osteoclasts (bone-resorbing cells). The lacunae are caused by the erosion of bone by osteoclast enzymes. These lacunae are seen on the surface of bone undergoing resorption. The scanning electron microscope reveals that these lacunae are shallow, irregularly shaped troughs, indicating the osteoclast activity and mobility during active resorption.

****

Q5) Haversian system

Q) Haversian canal

Q) Osteon

Answer – The basic building block of bone is the osteon, also known as the Haversian system.

- Bone's concentric layers are developed around a central vascular canal, called as Haversian canal. The concentric lamellae and Haversian canal collectively constitute the Osteon or Haversian system.

- In histologic section, an osteon is a long, cylindrical structure that runs parallel to the bone's long axis. Each osteon may have up to 20 concentric lamellae. A cement line [called reversal line] delineates the haversian systems. This line is strongly basophilic and may contain little or no collagen.

- Adjacent Haversian canals are connected by Volkmann canals. These canals house blood vessels, establishing a dense vascular network within the bone.

- Osteocytes are present in lacunae located at junctions of concentric lamellae. The canaliculi of the osteocytes radiate towards the Haversian canal. This connection mechanism will facilitate the exchange of nutrients and waste with the blood vessels present in the canal. Also adjacent osteocytes interconnect with each other by their processes.

- Interstitial lamellae fill the space between adjacent haversian systems.

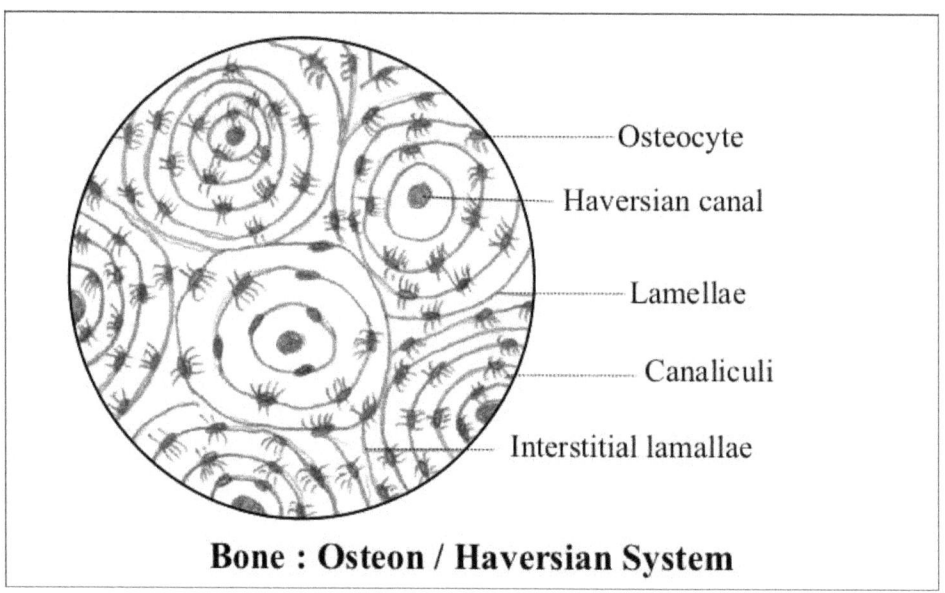

Bone : Osteon / Haversian System

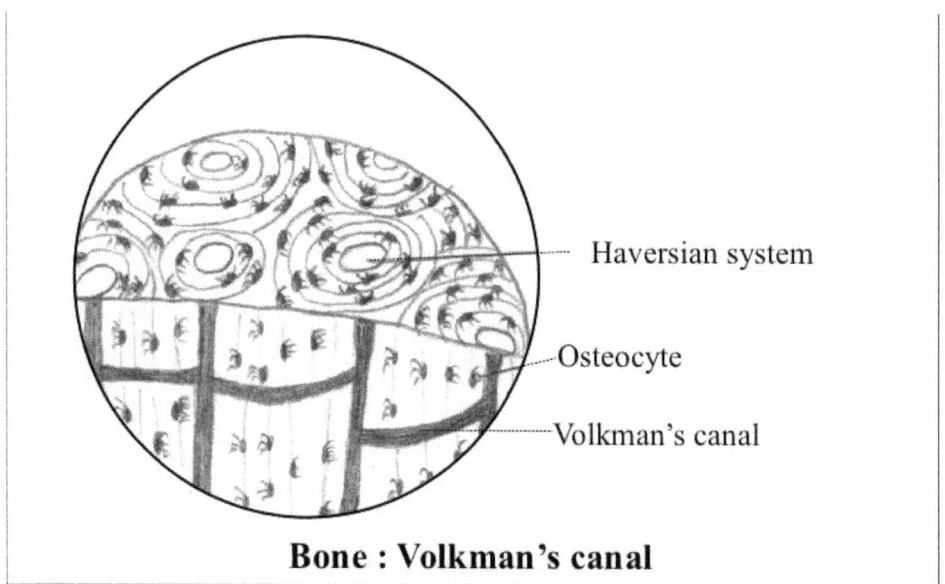

Bone : Volkman's canal

****

Q6) Osteoblasts.

Answer – The mononuclear cells called osteoblasts are in charge of creating and secreting the organic matrix that makes up bones. They also produce the bone matrix's collagenous and non-collagenous proteins.

- Osteoblasts are derived from osteoprogenitor cells present in bone marrow. The periosteum functions as a crucial reservoir of osteoblasts, specifically during childhood or following a bone fracture.
- They have an average life span of three months.

Morphology

- Osteoblasts are located on the surface of newly formed or remodeled bone.
- Active osteoblasts are plump, cuboidal, basophilic cells. Nucleus is situated eccentrically i.e. away from the bony surface. They have well-developed organelles associated with protein synthesis that include rER, ribosomes and mitochondria. Blueish hue of the cell is due to abundant rough endoplasmic reticulum.
- Inactive osteoblasts are flat with minimal synthetic organelles. They are termed as lining cells.
- Osteoblasts contact one another and the underlying osteocytes through their cytoplasmic processes thus maintaining cell-to-cell contact.

Functions of osteoblasts

- Osteoblasts primary function is the formation of new bone.
- It is essential for the mineralization of osteoid.
- Regulates bone remodeling (remodeling = sequential bone removal and deposition) and mineral metabolism.
- They identify and convey the resorptive signal to the osteoclast.

Fate of osteoblasts

Osteoblasts could have one of four distinct fates……

- May undergo apoptosis (programmed cell death).
- Get embedded into the bone it produces (osteocytes).
- They may differentiate into cells that form chondroid bone.
- They may transform to inactive osteoblasts and persist on the surface as bone lining cells.

****

Q7) Osteocytes.

Answer – Osteoblasts after producing the extracellular matrix of bone get entrapped within that matrix they have secreted. These entrapped osteoblasts and are now called osteocytes.

- The quantity of osteoblasts that transform into osteocytes is dependent upon the rate of bone deposition. The faster the bone production, the greater the quantity of osteocytes.
- Average life span of osteocytes is 25 years which is more than that of osteoblasts (only three months in human bone).
- When ground sections are being prepared, osteocytes are removed, leaving vacant spaces that are filled with debris. It appears black when observed in transmitted light using a light microscope.
- They are present in space called *osteocytic lacuna.*

- ***Osteocytic canaliculi*** -- Narrow extensions/canals called canaliculi radiate from this lacuna. These canals contain processes of osteocytes. The canaliculi facilitate communication among nearby osteocytes, osteoblasts and bone lining cells on the surface. This connecting system helps to maintain bone integrity and vitality. Loss of such contacts may lead to sclerosis or even necrosis of the bone. The canaliculi facilitate the flow of nutrients, gasses and waste materials between osteocytes and blood arteries.
- Osteocytes are smaller in size with few organelles. They have elliptical body with oval nucleus surrounded by narrow rim of cytoplasm.

****

Q8) Osteoclast.

Answer -- "Osteoclast" is a Greek term meaning "bone and broken".

- A bone cell called an osteoclast breaks down the mineralized matrix to resorb bone.
- It is derived from fusion of mononuclear cells of blood.
- Osteoclasts with a greater number of nuclei resorb more bone than those with fewer nuclei.

Morphology

- Morphology of osteoclast is variable due to their motility.
- They are large multinucleated cells with 15-20 closely packed nuclei.
- It lies in resorption bays called Howship's lacunae.
- Its cytoplasm contains an enzyme, acid phosphatase in vesicles, which helps for bone resorption.
- Osteoclast cell membrane is thrown into folds (ruffled border) adjacent to the surface of the bone that is to be resorbed.
- Several mechanisms bind osteoclasts to the bone surface. Bone surface contains osteopontin as well as bone sialoprotein, which could promote osteoclast attachment and the creation of the sealing zone.

****

Q9) Functions of alveolar bone.

Answer – The alveolar bone is described as the portion of maxilla and mandible that constitutes and supports the dental sockets.

- Houses the root/roots of the teeth.
- Attaches the teeth firmly to the bone. This firm anchorage is brought about by Sharpey's fibers which are inserted into the cementum at one end and the alveolar bone proper at the other end.
- Helps tooth movement for proper occlusion.
- Absorbs and distributes occlusal force that is generated while chewing.

- Serves as an outlet for the entrance of blood vessels and nerves to PDL.
- Houses and protects growing permanent tooth buds.
- Supports primary teeth.
- Facilitates the smooth eruption of both primary and permanent dentition.

Q10) Theories of mineralization

Answer – *There are three theories of mineralization.*

a) Alkaline phosphatase theory.
b) Nucleation theory.
c) Matrix vesicle theory.

ALKALINE PHOSPHATASE THEORY

- *Alkaline phosphatase* is an enzyme stored in the matrix vesicles in the cytoplasm of hard tissue-forming cells i.e. chondrocytes, osteoblasts and odontoblasts. It buds off from the cell membrane. This enzyme takes part in the calcification process by breaking down various substrates containing organic phosphates thereby increasing local phosphate ion concentration.
- Alkaline phosphatase enzyme breaks down inhibitors of hydroxyapatite crystal formation. It also initiates and promotes the growth of hydroxyapatite crystals by providing inorganic phosphates.

NUCLEATION THEORY

- This hypothesis is predicated on the principle of seeding or epitaxy (= growth of crystal).
- The theory suggests that a nucleus forms near collagen, which facilitates the accumulation of Ca+ and phosphate ions from the surrounding fluids. Hydroxyapatite crystals subsequently increase in size by the incorporation of these ions.

MATRIX VESICLE THEORY

- Matrix vesicles are tiny membrane-bound entities located freely within the cytoplasm.
- These matrix vesicles bud from the cells namely osteoblasts, chondrocytes and odontoblasts and provide a microenvironment for initial mineralization.
- Matrix vesicles are abundant in phospholipids and exhibit a strong affinity for calcium ions. Vesicles also include a protein known as annexins, which facilitates the incorporation of calcium ions into the vesicle. Matrix vesicles that contain accumulated calcium ions will promote the development of hydroxyapatite crystals. After attaining certain thickness, hydroxyapatite crystals in the matrix vesicle are released into the extracellular matrix. These released hydroxyapatite crystals serve as a template for further deposition of mineral crystals.

Q11) Describe bone formation.

Answer – Bone development transpires through two methods.

a) Endochondral / Intracartilaginous,
b) Intramembranous.

ENDOCHONDRAL / INTRACARTILAGINOUS BONE FORMATION

- Endochondral bone formation is a type of osteogenesis wherein a cartilaginous template is first laid down. This template is subsequently replaced by osseous tissue.
- *Site* – Ribs, mandibular articular extremity, cranial base.
- In the second month of development, mesenchymal cells condense and differentiate into chondroblasts (cartilage-forming cells). Chondroblasts secrete hyaline cartilage, leading to the development of a *hyaline cartilage model*. The perichondrium that envelops this model is made up of an outer fibrous layer and an internal chondrogenic layer. Because of the avascular environment at this point, no osteoblasts differentiate from the inner chondrogenic layer. To form a dense fibrous sheath, fibroblasts in the outer fibrous layer produce collagen. The length of the cartilage model increases through cellular division and matrix synthesis, while the breadth expands due to the deposition of new matrix at the model's periphery. This is brought about by chondroblasts originating from the perichondrium.
- Changes begin in the midsection of the cartilage model. Capillaries grow into the perichondrium thus increasing the nutrition supply. This promotes the development of osteoblasts from the perichondrium's inner layer. These osteoblasts then secrete a thin collar of bone matrix around the midsection of the cartilage model. The perichondrium will now be referred to as *periosteum* as its inner layer cells form bone. Later resorption of cartilage matrix occurs due to the action of chondroclasts. The cartilage which is weakened by disintegration is firmly held by the bone collar that has already formed
- Infiltration of periosteal capillaries and osteogenic cells in the cartilage model's central region, results in the formation of a structure called *periosteal bud*. This invasion commences the formation of a primary ossification center. The periosteal bud contains osteogenic cells. These cells transform into osteoblasts and lay down bone matrix over the residual cartilage thus forming cancellous bone.
- As the primary ossification center enlarges, osteoclasts resorb the newly developed spongy bone to create a medullary cavity within the bone's central region. Hematopoietic stem cells infiltrate the medullary cavity.

INTRAMEMBRANOUS BONE FORMATION

- Intramembranous ossification involves the direct development of bone within a fibrous membrane.
- E.g. -- flat bones of skull, clavicles.
- At the site where the bone is to develop, there ismesenchymal connective tissue havingstellate-shaped cells that are widely separated, but interconnected by their cytoplasmic processes. Osteogenesis begins at the center of this region. Stellate-shaped mesenchymal cells transform

into round cells and convert into osteoblasts. These osteoblasts release the organic matrix of bone. When these cells aresurroundedby bone matrix, they are referred to as osteocytes. Calcification of the newly deposited bone matrix and adjacent collagen fibers begins soon.

- The newly created bone matrix exhibits uneven spicule shape morphology. It progressively enlarges by anastomosing with adjacent spicules to create a structure known as trabeculae of woven bone. On the outer surface of this newly formed woven bone, condensation of vascularized mesenchyme leads to the formation of periosteum.
- The trabeculae deeper to the periosteum thicken, and form a collar of woven bone that is subsequently replaced by mature lamellar bone. Internally, spongy bone remains and its vascular tissue transforms into red marrow.
- During the transformation of cancellous bone into compact bone, numerous slender canals lined with osteogenic cells are created. These canals contain blood arteries that were formerly located in cancellous bone. As growth continues, successive layers of bone lamellae are deposited around the central cavity, resulting in the construction of an osteon or Haversian system.

****

Q11) Bundle bone.

Answer – Refer to section 'bundle bone' in short notes Q3 in chapter 'Bone'

****

MAXILLARY SINUS

SHORT NOTES

Q1) Histology of maxillary sinus.

Answer -- Maxillary sinus is a pneumatic space or air-filled space present in the body of maxilla.

HISTOLOGY

Histologically, 3 layers are seen......
- Epithelial layer.
- Basal lamina.
- Subepithelial layer including the periosteum.

EPITHELIUM

▶ The maxillary sinus is lined by pseudostratified ciliated columnar epithelium. The epithelium also contains basal cells, columnar non-ciliated cells, and mucous-secreting goblet cells.

▶ Ciliated cells comprise a nucleus, mitochondria, and vesicles containing enzymes. Ciliary microtubules are located in the top region of the cell. Beating of the cilia pushes the mucous on the epithelial surface to move from the maxillary sinus towards the nasal cavity.

▶ Goblet cells are flask-shaped cells. They exhibit distinctive property of a secretory cell, characterized by a plentiful of rER, golgi apparatus and mitochondria. Zymogen granules that contain mucopolysaccharides are present in golgi complex. These granules are transported from the Golgi complex to the cell apex and released on epithelial surface by exocytosis.

▶ The minor salivary glands located in the subepithelial layer of the sinus secrete their products through excretory ducts onto epithelial surface.

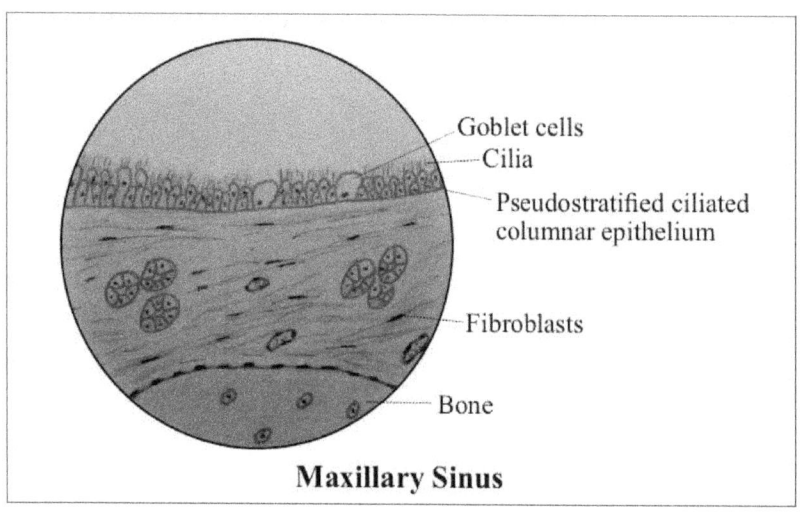

Maxillary Sinus

****

Q2) Functions of maxillary sinus.

Answer – Maxillary sinus is a pneumatic space or air-filled space present in the body of maxilla. It performs the following functions……

- ▶ Gives resonance to the voice.
- ▶ Reduces weight of the skull.
- ▶ Produces bactericidal enzymes.
- ▶ Protects brain and eye ball against exposure to cold air.
- ▶ Help in absorbing the shock of blows to the face.
- ▶ Insulation, humidifying and warming of inspired air.
- ▶ Contributes to the sense of smell (olfaction).

****

Q3) Maxillary sinus.

Answer–Write short notes Q1 and Q2 from chapter 'Maxillary sinus'

****

ORAL MUCOUS MEMBRANE

MAIN QUESTIONS

Q1) Classify oral mucosa. Describe the histology of keratinized stratified squamous epithelium.

Answer – The term 'oral mucous membrane' also known as 'oral mucosa' describes the moist lining of the mouth.

CLASSIFICATION OF ORAL MUCOSA

Oral mucous membrane is classified into three types based upon its functions......

Masticatory Mucosa: Comprises 25% of the total mucosa. The main mucosa that contacts food during mastication. It comprises of gingiva and hard palate. It is firmly attached to the surrounding bone and immovable. It is generally keratinized.

Lining / Reflecting Mucosa: Constitutes 60% of total mucosa. It plays no role in mastication. It involves the floor of the mouth, ventral tongue, alveolar mucosa, buccal mucosa, lips and soft palate. It is soft and flexible. It lacks keratin.

Specialized Mucosa: Comprises 15% of the total oral mucosa. It is present on the dorsal surface of the tongue.

Oral mucosa may also be classified as......

Keratinized areas ---------- Masticatory mucosa and vermilion border of lip
Nonkeratinized areas ------ Lining mucosa
Specialized mucosa -------- Dorsum of tongue

HISTOLOGY

- There are two kinds of oral mucous membrane epithelium: stratified squamous keratinized and non-keratinized.
- Stratified squamous keratinized epithelium can be classified as either orthokeratinized or parakeratinized.
- *In keratinized epithelium, the cells are arranged in four cell layers and these layers are named based on their morphologic appearance. Each cell is a part of each layer at different times. A solitary cell post-mitosis may persist within the basal layer and continue division when needed. Alternatively, it may migrate to the highest levels, during which significant biochemical and morphological changes occur. This is termed differentiation. When it reaches the surface, it is exfoliated or desquamated. The process by which cells migrate from the basal layer to the surface is referred to as "maturation."*

Four layers in keratinized epithelium from bottom to top are…..

1) Basal layer [Stratum basale]
2) Spinous layer [Stratum spinosum]
3) Granular layer [Stratum granulosum]
4) Cornified layer [Stratum corneum]

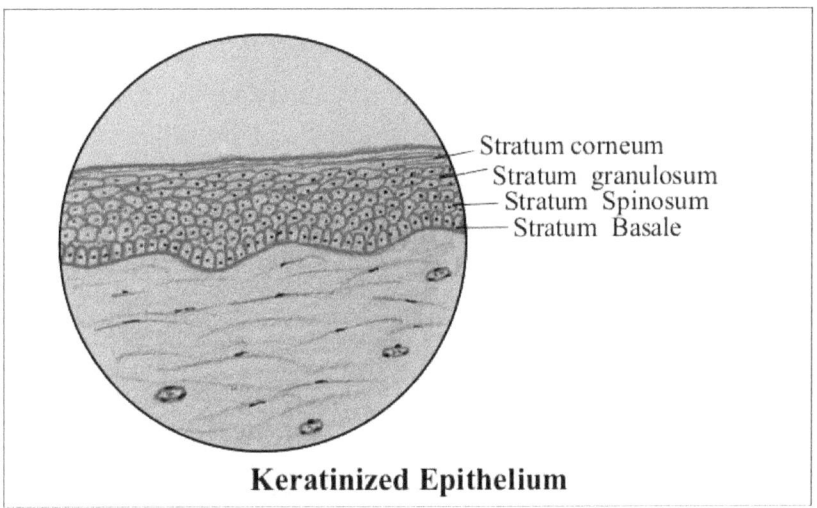

Keratinized Epithelium

Stratum basale

- The cells in this layer lie over the basement membrane.
- This layer constitutes of a single layer of cuboidal cells that go through mitosis to produce new cells.
- Mitotic figures may also be seen in the upper spinous layer. Hence both basal and parabasal layers (upper spinous layer) are called stratum germinativum.
- Basal cells consist of two populations: serrated cells and nonserrated cells.
- **Serrated cells** – Serrated cells consist of a single layer of cuboidal cells with cytoplasmic processes extending from the basal surface toward the underlying connective tissue. They are heavily packed with tonofilaments for the purpose of attachment.
- **Nonserrated cells** -- Non-serrated cells consist of slowly proliferating stem cells that preserve the genetic material of the tissue.

Junctions between oral epithelial cells

a) Desmosomal junction between the cells,
b) Hemidesmosomal junction between the cell and basement membrane.

Stratum spinosum

- This is the second layer lying over the stratum basale.

- Cells of spinous layer are polyhedral in shape and larger than the basal cells. Shrinkage caused during tissue processing separates the spinous cells from adjacent cells except at the point of desmosomal contact. This gives a spiny appearance to the layer, thus the name. Among the 4 layers, the spinous cells exhibit significant activity in protein synthesis.

Stratum granulosum

- This is the third layer lying over the stratum spinosum.
- Cells in the granulosum layer are flattened and broader than the spinous cells. This layer is designated as such because of the basophilic keratohyalin granules presence within the cells. The cells are tightly adhered to one another. Tonofilaments are dense in quantity. Nuclei of these cells show signs of degenerationand pyknosis. The cells still synthesize proteins.
- A lamellar granule, sometimes referred to as a keratinosome, Odland body, or membrane-coating granule, is observed in upper spinous and granular layers. These are in fact lamellated glycolipids.

Stratum corneum

- This is the topmost layer lying above stratum granulosum layer.
- The orthokeratinized epithelium consists of keratinized squamae that are bigger and more flattened than the underlying cells. Nuclei, keratohyalin granules and cellular organelles are eliminated. The cells are dehydrated and tightly adhered to one another. It encompasses a larger region than the basal cell from whence it originated. It does not produce protein.
- Until desquamation takes place, the cells in parakeratinized epithelium retain pyknotic condensed nuclei and other partially destroyed organelles.
- Ultrastructurally, the cells are seen to contain densely packed tonofilaments.

Keratinocytes and Non-keratinocytes

Both keratinized and non-keratinized epithelium comprises two categories of cells.

- *Keratinocytes* –The cells of stratum basale, stratum granulosum, stratum spinosum, and stratum corneum are keratinocytes. They undergo mitosis, maturation and desquamation. Their size increases from the basal layer to the superficial layer.
- *Nonkeratinocytes*– These are a small population of cells that are present between the keratinocytes. They do not experience mitosis, maturation or desquamation. They are not organized in layers and do not establish desmosomal connections with neighboring keratinocytes. They possess dendrites or processes. They are distinctly visible in H and E stained sections and are recognized only through specific stains. They originate from the neural crest or bone marrow and migrate to the mouth epithelium. Non keratinocytes family includes ---melanocytes, Langerhanscells, merkelcells, lymphocytes.
- Refer to short notes Q13 in chapter "Oral mucous membrane".

****

Q2) Classify oral mucosa. Describe the histology of non-keratinized stratified squamous epithelium.

Answer – 'Oral mucous membrane' or 'oral mucosa' refers to the moist lining of the mouth.

CLASSIFICATION

- Refer to section 'Classification of oral mucosa' in main question Q1 in chapter "Oral mucous membrane".

HISTOLOGY OF NON KERATINIZED EPITHELIUM / MUCOSA

- Epithelium of oral mucous membrane may be stratified squamous keratinized or non-keratinized types.
- Non-keratinized epithelium is thicker than keratinized epithelium.
- Non-keratinized epithelium is distinguished from keratinized epithelium by its lack of cornified surface.
- *In nonkeratinized epithelium, the cells are arranged in three cell layers and these layers are named based on their morphologic appearance. Each cell is a part of each layer at different times. A solitary cell post-mitosis may persist in the basal layer and continue division when needed. Alternatively, it may migrate to the top levels, during which significant biochemical and morphological changes occur. This is referred to as differentiation. Upon reaching the surface, it undergoes desquamation. 'Maturation' is a term to describe the mechanism of cell migration from the basal layer to the surface.*
- **Three layers in non keratinized epithelium from bottom to top are…..**

    1) Basal layer [Stratum basale]
    2) Intermediate layer [Stratum intermedium]
    3) Superficial layer [Stratum superficiale]

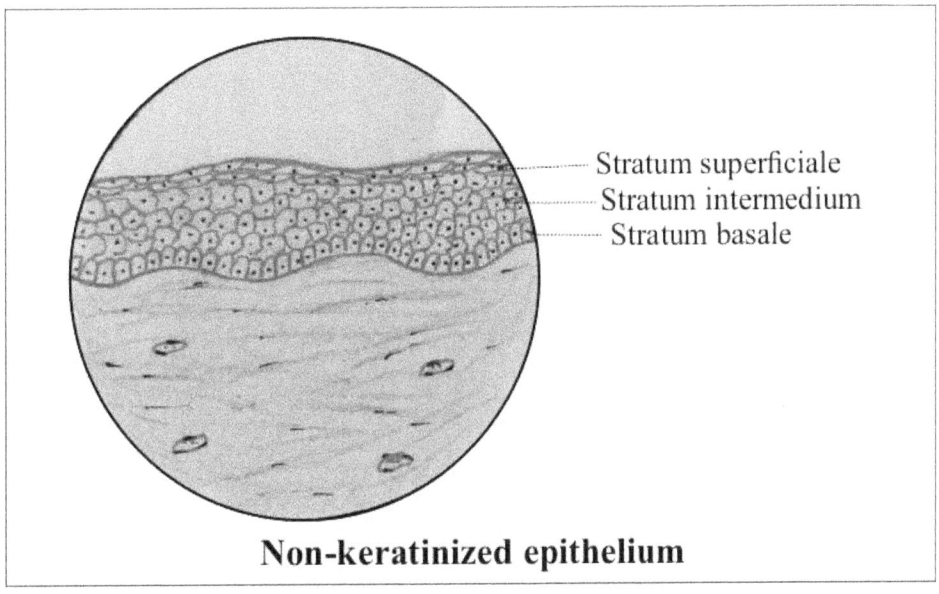

Non-keratinized epithelium

Stratum basale

- The cells in this layer lie over the basement membrane.
- The basal layer involves single layer of cuboidal cells that undergo mitosis to generate new cells. Mitosis is more prevalent than in the keratinized mucosa.

Junctions between oral epithelial cells

a) Desmosomal junction between the cells,
b) Hemidesmosomal junction between the cell and basement membrane.

Stratum intermedium

- This is the second layer lying over the stratum basale.
- In contrast to the stratum spinosum cells in keratinized mucosa, the stratum intermedium cells are bigger and much closely connected by desmosomal connections, lacking intercellular space. Hence spinous appearance is not seen in stratum intermedium layer.

Stratum superficiale

- This is the topmost layer lying above stratum intermedium.
- Cells in this layer are flat and contain nuclei. These cells are shed off.

****

Q3) Describe the macroscopy and microscopy of masticatory mucosa.

Answer -- 'Oral mucous membrane' or 'oral mucosa' refers to the moist lining of the mouth. The masticatory mucosa comprises the hard palate along with gingiva. It is keratinized.

HARD PALATE

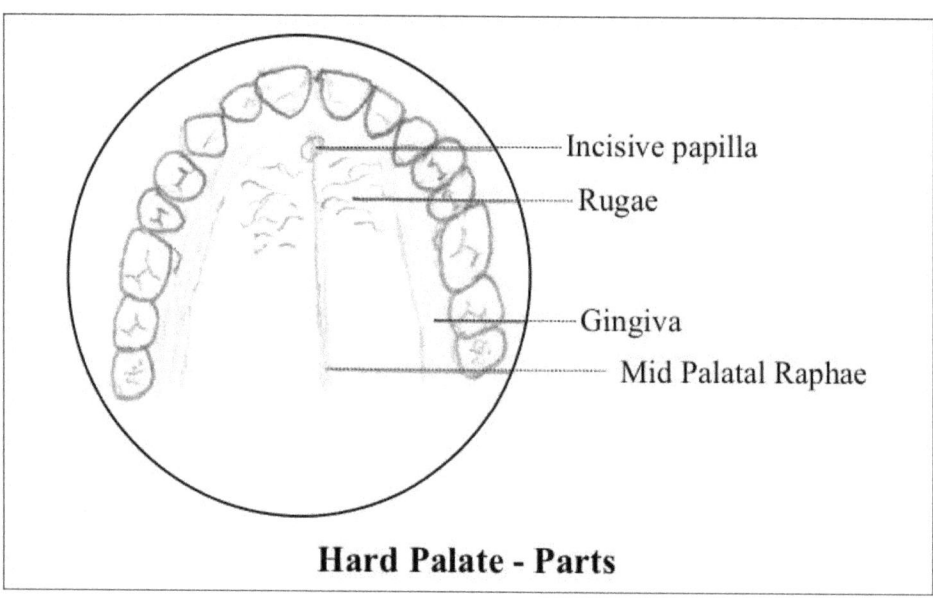

Hard Palate - Parts

Macroscopy

- Hard palate's mucous membrane is firmly fixed to the underlying periosteum covering the bone and hence is immovable.
- Its colour is pink like gingiva.
- Irregular, thick, mucous membranes asymmetric ridges located in the anterior area of the hard "palate are referred to as palatine rugae. They extend laterally from the mid-palatine raphe and the incisive papilla.

Various zones can be noted

- *Gingival region* – adjacent to the teeth.
- *Palatine raphe* – Extending posteriorly from the incisive papilla along the midline.
- *Fatty zone* – anterolateral area between raphe and gingiva.
- *Glandular zone* – posterolateral area between raphe and gingiva.

Microscopy / Histology

Epithelium

Refer section 'Histology of keratinized epithelium' in main question Q1 in chapter "Oral mucous membrane"

Lamina propria

- The lamina propria is denser in the anterior area of the hard palate compared to the posterior area. It possesses several elongated connective tissue papillae.
- Regions in the hard palate vary depending upon the structure of submucosa.
- *Incisive papilla* – This region consists of dense connective tissue with nasopalatine ducts lined by stratified or pseudostratified columnar epithelium. Small mucous glands open into their ducts. Concentrically grouped cells which frequently undergo keratinization are noted in the lamina propria along the fusion line of palatine processes. These are remnants of epithelium (epithelial pearls).
- *Palatine rugae* -- It consists of dense fibrous connective tissue.

Submucosa

- The submucous layer is absent peripherally where the hard palate merges with the gingiva. Below the epithelium lies only the periosteum and lamina propria. Submucosa is also absent along the mid-palatine raphe.
- The submucosa in the anterolateral and posterolateral regions is separated into irregular, intercommunicating compartments of varying sizes. The anterior region is occupied by adipose tissue, whereas the posterior region contains small salivary glands.

- Anterior palatine nerves and vessels pass at the junction of the alveolar process and the horizontal plate of the hard palate.

GINGIVA

Macroscopy

- The gingiva runs from the dentinogingival junction to the alveolar mucosa.
- The mucogingival junction separates the gingiva from the alveolar mucosa. This demarcation is clinically seen as the intersection between pale pink gingiva and bright pink alveolar mucosa. On the lingual aspect of the lower jaw, a demarcation line may be seen between gingiva and floor of the mouth. The distinction between gingiva and palatal mucosa on the hard palate is unclear.

Colour

- Normal colour of gingiva is pink. At times, it may exhibit a shade of gray.
- Colour depends on whether it is keratinized or non-keratinized, thickness, and also on the amount of pigmentation.

Parts of gingiva

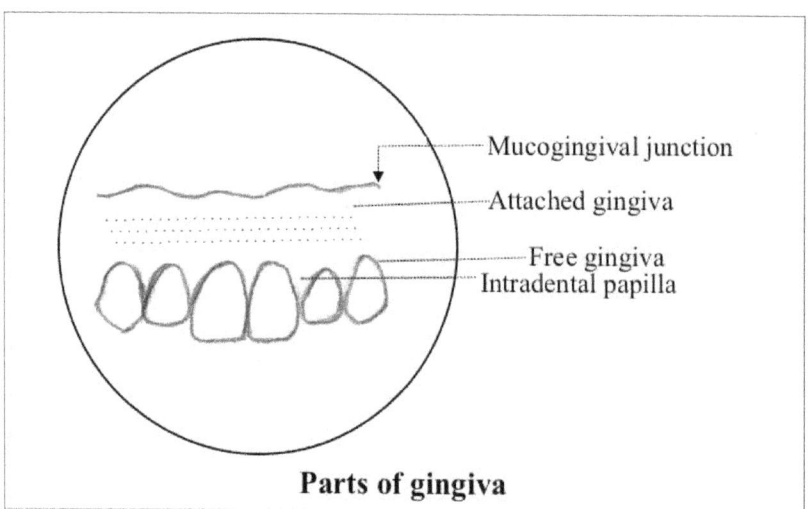

Parts of gingiva

Gingiva can be divided into three parts

a) Free gingiva
b) Attached gingiva
c) Interdental papilla

Free gingiva

- Free gingiva is separated from the attached gingiva by a line called *free gingival groove*.

- Clinically although not visible, it can be seen as a shallow V-shaped notch in the histologic sections. It is approximately 0.5 - 1.5mm from the gingival margin. It may be located at the level or a little below the base of gingival sulcus.

Attached gingiva

- The width of attached gingiva measures approximately 4-6 mm.
- It is delineated from the alveolar mucosa by the mucogingival groove.
- It is attached to the tooth by junctional epithelium.
- Attached gingiva is characterized by stippled surface. Clinically stippling can be seen as small pits or depression on the surface of healthy gingiva. This could be a functional adaptation of gingiva to withstand mechanical stress. The absence of stippling signifies edema and inflammation of the gingiva (gingivitis). The degree of stippling varies between individuals, age and sex. Men show more stippling than women. Histologically, the epithelium in the stippled areas appears to be elevated with shallow depressions in-between.

Interdental papilla

- The interdental papilla is the portion of the gingiva that occupies the space between two neighboring teeth.
- It appears triangular in shape from the buccal or lingual side. In a three-dimensional perspective, the posterior teeth's interdental papilla exhibits a 'tent' shape, while that of the anterior teeth has a 'pyramidal' form. This is due to the narrow contact point in the anterior teeth and the wide contact area in posterior teeth.
- Melanin pigmentation is more at the papilla's base.
- In the interdental papilla of posterior teeth, the oral and vestibular corners are high, creating with a valley or depression in the center. This middle concave region is situated below the contact area and is referred to as the *col. The col is enveloped by a thin, nonkeratinized epithelium, rendering it more susceptible to periodontal disease.*

Microscopy / Histology

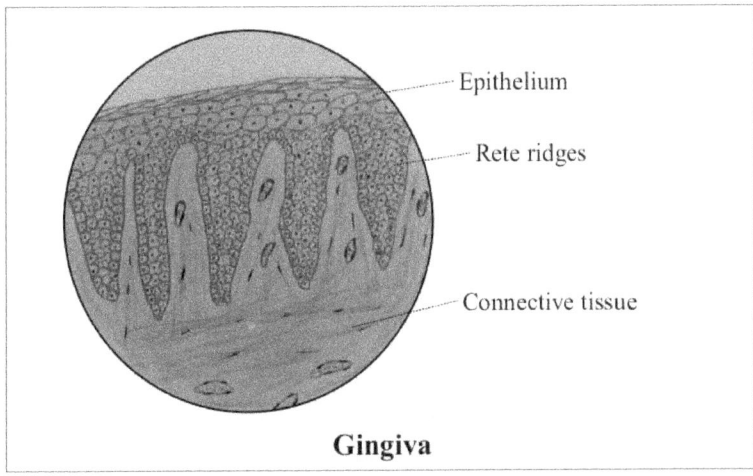

Gingiva

Epithelium

- The epithelium of gingiva is parakeratinized in seventy-five percent of instances, orthokeratinized in fifteen percent and nonkeratinized in ten-percent.
- Rete ridges or rete pegs are irregular, long, numerous and slender.
- Refer to section 'Histology of keratinized epithelium' in main question Q1 in chapter "Oral mucous membrane".

Lamina propria

- The lamina propria shows dense connective tissue and lacks significant blood arteries.
- Connective tissue papillae in gingiva are irregular, elongated, slender and abundant. These papillae facilitate the clear distinction between gingiva and alveolar mucosa, wherein the papillae are relatively short and few.
- Few inflammatory cells can be seen.
- The gingiva lacks submucosa. It is firmly attached to periosteum that envelops the alveolar bone. Hence it is also cited as *mucoperiosteum*.
- The gingiva's lamina propria contains few principal fibers of the periodontal ligament, that helps the gingiva firmly adhere to the teeth.
- Refer to section 'Gingival fiber group' in main question Q1 in chapter 'Periodontal ligament'.

Apart from these the other fibers that run in the lamia propria of gingiva are

- Interdental fibers – These fibers connect buccal and lingual interdental papillae.
- Semicircular fibers – These fibers extend from the cementum on one side of the tooth, traverse the free gingiva and are inserted into the cementum on the opposing side.
- Vertical fibers -- These fibers originate from the alveolar mucosa or attachedgingiva, traverses upwards vertically to get inserted in the free gingiva or interdental papillae.
- Transgingival fibers–These fibers mingle with circular and semicircular fibers as they run from the cementum of one tooth to the adjacent tooth's marginal gingiva.

****

Q4) Discuss the histology of buccal mucosa.

Answer– 'Oral mucous membrane' or 'oral mucosa refers to the moist lining of the mouth. The buccal mucosa is categorized as lining mucosa and is non-keratinized.

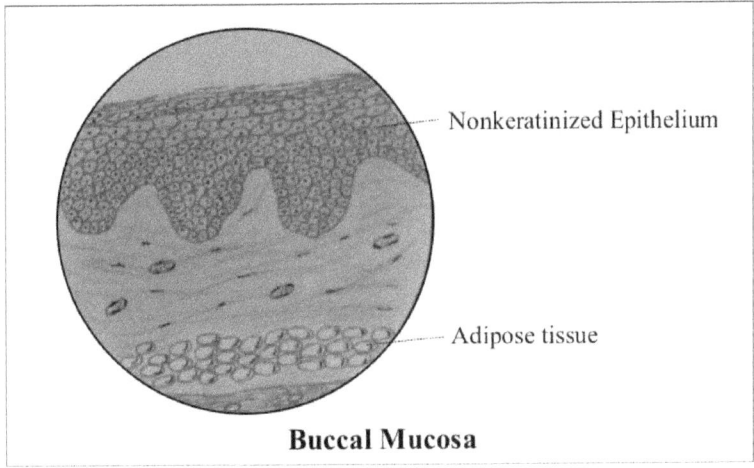

Buccal Mucosa

Epithelium

Refer section 'Histology of non keratinized epithelium' in main question Q2 in chapter "Oral mucous membrane"

Lamina propria

- It comprises dense fibrous connective tissue featuring irregular, short, wide papillae.

Submucosa

- The submucosa comprises dense bundles of collagen fibers, buccinator muscle and adipose tissue.

****

Q5) Discuss the histology of labial mucosa.

Answer– 'Oral mucous membrane' or 'oral mucosa' refers to the moist lining of the mouth. Labial mucosa is classified as lining mucosa and is non-keratinized.

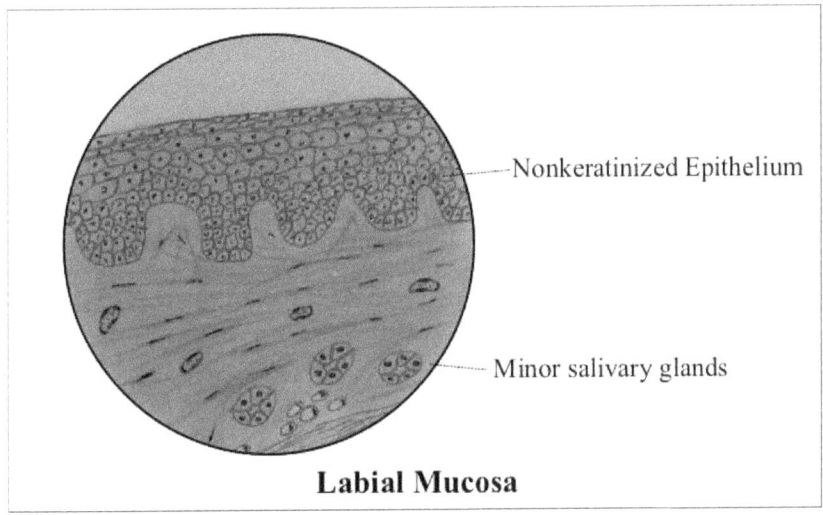

Labial Mucosa

Epithelium

Refer to section 'Histology of non keratinized epithelium' in main question Q2 in chapter "Oral mucous membrane".

Lamina propria

- The lamina propria comprises dense bundles of collagen fibers interspersed with short, irregular papillae.

Submucosa

- The submucosa comprises tight bundles of collagen fibers, orbicularis oris muscle and small salivary glands.

****

Q6) Describe in detail specialized mucosa.

Answer -- Specialized mucosa consists of the dorsal lingual mucosa and taste buds.

DORSAL LINGUAL MUCOSA

- The mucosa of the dorsal or superior surface of tongue is rough and irregular. It is divided into the anterior two-thirds (or body) and the posterior one-third (or base) by a V-shaped line known as the *sulcus terminalis*.
- The anterior section is referred to as the *'papillary portion'* because of the abundance of very fine, pointed, cone-shaped papillae. These papillae impart a velvety texture and appearance to the tongue.
- Posterior part is called *'lymphatic portion'* because of the presence of lymphoid tissue.
- Four varieties of papillae are observed on the dorsal side of tongue. These are...

    a) Filiform papillae
    b) Fungiform papillae
    c) Circumvallate papillae
    d) Foliate papillae

Filiform papillae

- Filiform papillae are many, slender, pointed, conical structures that gives a velvety texture to the surface.
- Site – They are found in the anterior part of tongue.
- These structures are enveloped by partially keratinized epithelium and contain a core of connective tissue.
- *They lack taste buds.*

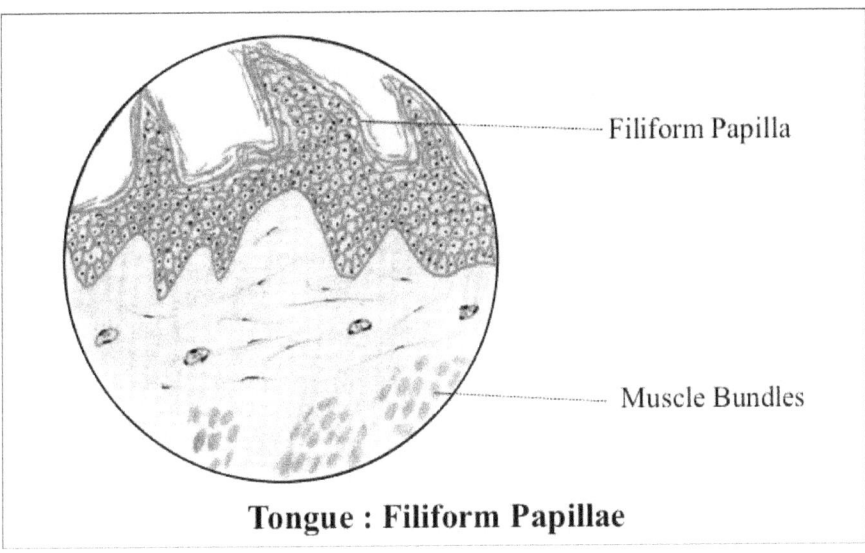

Tongue : Filiform Papillae

Fungiform papillae

- Fungiform means 'fungus-like' or 'mushroom-like'.
- These are isolated papillae interspersed between the filiform papillae.
- They are smooth, spherical formations that appear red due to a highly vascularized connective tissue core.
- It is bordered by a thin, nonkeratinized stratified squamous epithelium.
- They contain only few (1-3) taste buds.

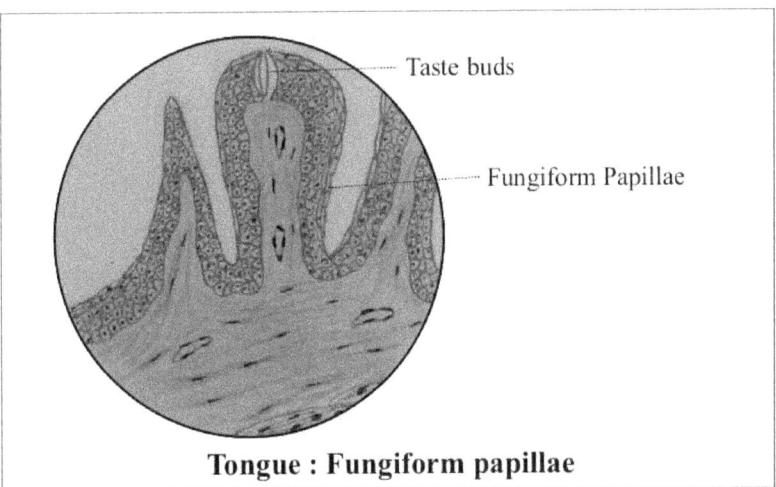

Tongue : Fungiform papillae

Circumvallate papillae

- Circumvallate means 'walled'.
- These are located anterior to the V-shaped terminal sulcus, present at the junction of the body and the tongue base.
- They are large and are 8-10 in number.
- They have a narrow base and do not protrude above the tongue surface.

- They are surrounded by a deep circular trough or sulcus. The ducts of small serous glands, known as *von Ebner's* glands, discharge into this trough and assist in the removal of soluble food material that has collected within the troughs.
- The epithelium on the lateral surface of this papilla has many taste buds.

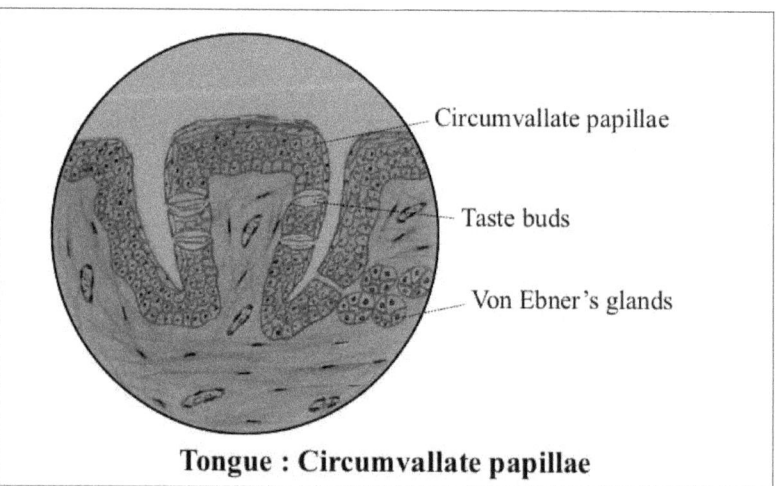

Tongue : Circumvallate papillae

Foliate papillae

- Foliate means 'Leaf-like'.
- They are distinct parallel fissures of varied lengths located on lateral margin of the posterior tongue and are readily identifiable.
- A limited number of taste buds are located in epithelium.
- Serous glands are located beneath the taste buds, facilitating the cleansing of the grooves.

TASTE BUDS

- Taste buds are specialized sensory organs that detect taste.
- They are little, ovoid, barrel-shaped intraepithelial structures.
- They run from basal lamina to the epithelial surface. A tiny aperture (taste pore) exists on the external surface. A taste bud may contain several taste pores. This pore opens into a constricted area bordered by the taste buds supporting cells. The peripheral supporting cells are organized resembling staves of a barrel. The inner supporting cells are small and have fusiform morphology. Neuroepithelial cells, which function as receptors for taste impulses are situated among the supporting cells.

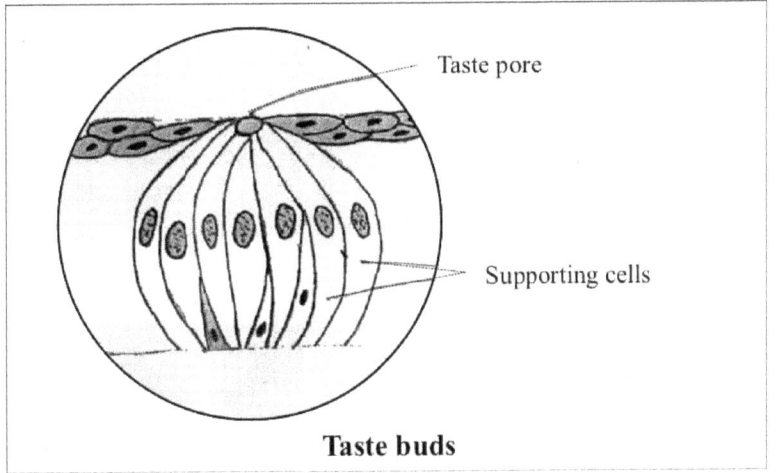

Taste buds

Site of taste buds

- Inner wall of the trough around the vallate papilla (numerous),
- In the folds of the foliate papilla,
- On the posterior surface of epiglottis,
- Some on the tip of fungiform papillae,
- Lateral border of tongue.

TASTE SENSATIONS

Tongue

Tip – sweet

Lateral part – salty, sour

Middle part – bitter

Papillae

Vallate – bitter

Foliate – sour

Fungiform – sweet (at the tip); salty (at the border)

Palate

Bitter and sour.

****

SHORT NOTES

Q1) Papillae of tongue.

Answer – Refer to section 'Dorsal lingual mucosa' in main question Q6 in chapter "Oral mucous membrane"

****

Q2) Filiform and fungiform papillae of tongue.

Answer – Refer to section 'Filiform and fungiform papillae of tongue' in main question Q6 in chapter "Oral mucous membrane".

****

Q3) Specialized mucosa

Q) Specialized oral mucosa.

Answer – Refer to main question Q6 in chapter "Oral mucous membrane".

****

Q4) Taste buds.

Answer – Refer to section 'Taste buds' in main question Q6 in chapter "Oral mucous membrane".

****

Q5) Masticatory mucosa.

Answer – Refer to main question Q3 in chapter "Oral mucous membrane".

****

Q6) Lining mucosa

Q) Lip mucosa.

Answer – Refer to main question Q4 in chapter "Oral mucous membrane".

****

Q7) Gingiva

Q) Histology of gingiva.

Answer -- Refer to section 'Gingiva' in main question Q3 in chapter "Oral mucous membrane".

****

Q8) Keratinized epithelium

Q) Keratinized mucosa.

Answer – Refer to section 'Histology of keratinized epithelium / Keratinized mucosa' in main question Q1 in chapter "Oral mucous membrane".

***

Q9) Stratum basale and stratum spinosum.

Answer – Refer to section 'Stratum basale and Stratum spinosum' in 'Histology of keratinized epithelium' in main question Q1 in chapter "Oral mucous membrane".

***

Q10) Gingival COL.

Answer -- In the posterior teeth, the oral and vestibular interdental papillae are high, creating a valley or depression in the center. This middle concave region is situated beneath the contact area and is referred to as the *col. Col epithelium is similar to junctional epithelium.* The col is covered by thin, non-keratinized epithelium, rendering it more susceptible to periodontal disease. Increased proneness could be due to the fact that gingivitis in the interdental area is more due to the tooth contour which favors food accumulation.

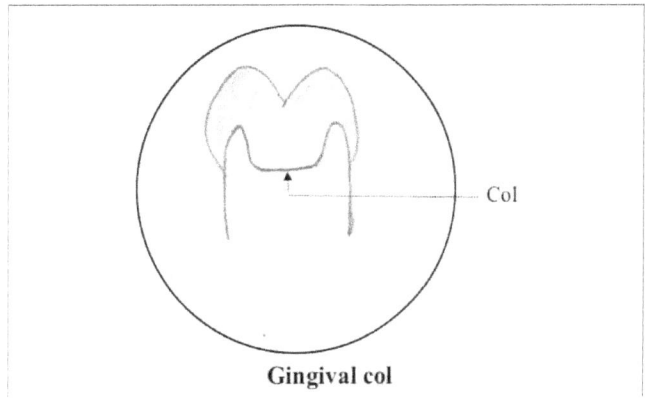

Gingival col

***

Q11) Vermilion zone of lip

Q) Vermilion border of lip

Answer – The vermilion zone of the lip is a mucocutaneous junction that marks the transition between the skin of the lip and its mucous membrane. The line between the skin and the vermilion zone is referred to as the *vermilion border*. It is only observed in humans. This line is clearly defined in youth and diffused in those exposed to UV radiation.

HISTOLOGY

Skin of lip

- The lip's skin is enveloped by slightly thick, keratinized epithelium with broad stratum corneum.
- Connective tissue papillae are few and short.
- Adnexal structures like sweat glands and sebaceous glands are found near hair follicles.

Mucous membrane of lip

- The mucous membrane of the lip is made up of stratified squamous keratinized epithelium. Connective tissue papillae are elongated. The lamina propria contains large capillary loops.
- Lamina propria does not contain salivary glands and hence it dries and cracks in winter.
- Fibers of the orbicularis oris muscle are observed in the submucosa.
- In the inner aspect of lip, vermilion zone continues as labial mucosa which can be easily identified by its thicker nonkeratinized epithelium.

What gives red colour to the vermillion zone?

- Epithelium of vermilion zone is thin and mildly keratinized.
- Connective tissue papillae are abundant, elongated and penetrate deeply into the epithelium. It contains extensive capillary loops that provide the red color of blood to the vermilion zone.

****

Q12) Gingival sulcus

Q) Gingival crevice

Answer –

- The gingival sulcus or crevice is a space located between the inner aspect of the gingiva and the tooth surface.
- It persists around the tooth's circumference.
- It runs from free gingival border to the dentogingival junction.
- The epithelium of gingival sulcus" (sulcular epithelium) is nonkeratinized. The epithelium is thinner than in gingiva. It does not have epithelial rete ridges but forms a smooth interface with lamina propria. The epithelium is continuing with the gingival epithelium and junctional epithelium.
- The sulcus contains fluid (gingival crevicular fluid / GCF) that has passed from the junctional epithelium, desquamated epithelial cells of the sulcular and junctional epithelia and inflammatory cells.

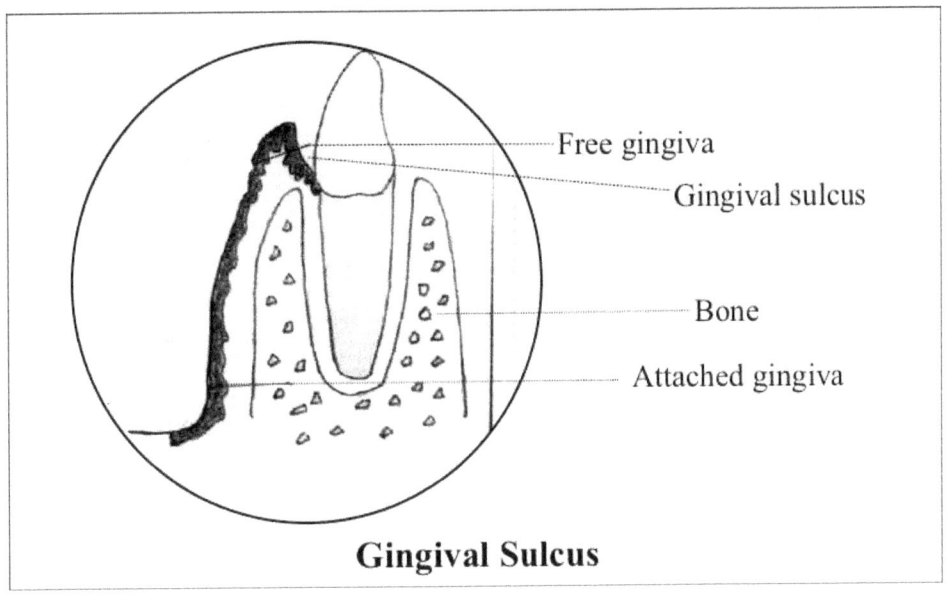

Gingival Sulcus

Depth of gingival sulcus

- Depth of gingival sulcus is variable. 2mm depth is considered normal.
- Approximately it is till the level of free gingival groove (in health).
- Depth of 3mm or more is regarded as pathologic (periodontal disease). This deepened sulcus is termed a 'periodontal pocket'.

Formation of gingival sulcus

- During tooth eruption, there is fusion of the reduced enamel epithelium that covers the crown of newly formed tooth and oral epithelium. The cells in the centre of this fused epithelia degenerate due to lack of nutrition and thus a perforation is created which creates a passage for the crown to emerge into the oral cavity. The portion of the enamel that has not yet erupted still has reduced enamel epithelium attached to it.
- The REE progressively gets shorter as the tooth eruption progresses, and a shallow groove known as the gingival sulcus forms between the gingiva and the tooth's surface. The entire tooth is surrounded by this groove.

****

Q13) Non-keratinocytes.

Answer – Non-keratinocytes comprise a small population of cells interspersed between the keratinocytes in the basal layer of the epithelium. They do not undergo mitosis, maturation and desquamation. They don't form a layer and do not have contact with the keratinocytes next to them. They have dendrites or processes and appear as clear cells in H and E stained sections. They are identified only by special stains. They move from the bone marrow or neural crest to the oral epithelium.

Non keratinocytes in the oral epithelium are

- Melanocytes,
- Langerhans cells,
- Merkel cells,
- Lymphocytes.

MELANOCYTES

- These are the cells located in epithelium's basal layer and are responsible for synthesizing melanin, a pigment that imparts color to the mucosa.
- They appear clear cells in H & E stain. With silver stain, their dendritic (spider-like) appearance can be seen. Hence melanocytes are additionally called as *clear cells / dendritic cells.*
- Melanin synthesized in melanocytes is carried by their dendritic processes to neighboring basal keratinocytes, which accumulate them as *melanosomes.*
- Melanin pigment leaked into the connective tissue is engulfed by macrophages *[called 'melanophages'].*
- Melanocyte number varies in different regions. The degree of pigmentation is due to the activity of the melanocytes is not related to their number.

LANGERHANS CELL

- Langerhans cells are also clear or dendritic cells observed in the epithelium's upper layers.
- They are of hematopoietic origin.
- The cell has characteristic rod-like granules *[Birbeck granules].*
- They enter the epithelium through lamina propria.

Functions

- They are associated with immunologic response. They pick up antigens and present them to the lymphocytes.

MERKEL CELL

- Merkels cells are also observed in the basal layer of the oral epithelium.

- They are of neural crest origin.
- They are considered to be specialized neural receptors responsive to pressure.
- Typically observed in masticatory mucosa and absent in lining mucosa.
- They are non dendritic i.e. do not have dendritic processes.
- The cells contain characteristic electron-dense granules situated at the side of cytoplasm in contact with the neural tissue. Function of these granules is not known.

****

Q14) Age changes in the oral mucosa.

Answer -- The following changes can be seen in oral mucosa with ageing…..

Oral mucosa – Oral mucosa becomes smooth and dry. This could be because of the thinning of the epithelium. Epithelial-connective tissue junction becomes smooth due to flattening of the rete ridges. Dryness is due to decrease in salivary secretion. Patients may complain of dryness of mouth, burning sensation and altered taste. This could be also due to systemic disease and medication with ageing. Sebaceous glands (Fordyce's spots) may increase on the lip and buccal mucosa.

Tongue – Filiform papillae are reduced in number. The tongue exhibits a smooth and shiny appearance due to decrease in epithelial thickness. Reduction in filiform papillae makes the fungiform papillae more prominent. Varicose veins on ventral surface of the tongue are frequently observed and are referred to as lingual varices.

Minor salivary glands – They may show atrophy and fibrosis.

Lamina propria – Cell number decreases with age. Collagen content increases.

Langerhans cells – Number decreases with ageing, thereby leading to a decrease in cell-mediated immunity.

Nerves – As people age, they may gradually lose their sensation to mechanical, chemical and temperature stimuli as well as their ability to perceive taste.

****

Q15) Dento-gingival junction.

Q) Junctional epithelium.

Answer –The dentogingival junction refers to the connection between the tooth and the gingiva.

- The gingiva's epithelium that adheres to the tooth is referred to as junctional epithelium or attachment epithelium. This union is referred to as *epithelial attachment*.
- Junctional epithelium extends up to 2mm on the surface of the tooth and thereafter it continues upwards as the sulcular epithelium.

- The epithelium's attachment to the tooth is very firm. When gingiva is tried to detach from the tooth, the junctional epithelium tears but does not peel from the enamel surface.

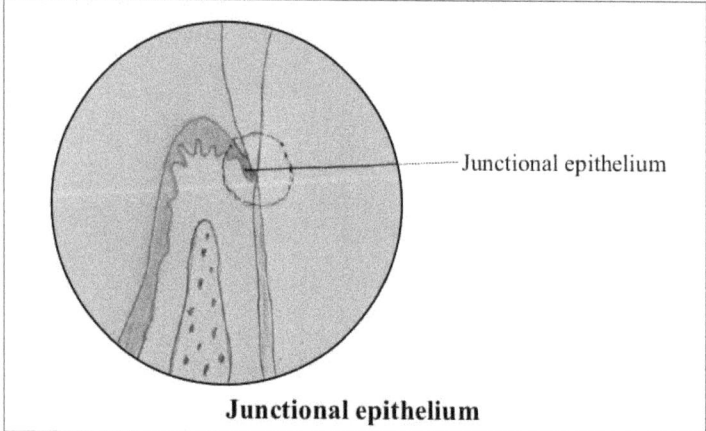

Junctional epithelium

- *Histology*-- Junctional epithelium is described as a no-differentiating, nonkeratinizing tissue. It is akin to the reduced enamel epithelium having a basal layer and multiple layers of flattened cells above which are parallel to the tooth surface. Large intercellular gap increases junctional epithelium permeability and lets neutrophils and gingival fluid enter the sulcus.
- *Clinical importance*– It represents a point of less resistance to mechanical forces and bacterial infiltration. Bacteria on the tooth surface produce toxins that initiate inflammation and damage this junction.

Development of dentogingival junction

- Upon the complete secretion of the enamel matrix, the ameloblasts deposit a thin membrane on the enamel surface (*primary enamel cuticle*) and subsequently diminish in size.
- The inner enamel epithelium, stratum intermedium and outer enamel epithelium constitute the *reduced enamel epithelium.* This envelops the entire enamel surface, extending to the CEJ and remains attached to the primary enamel cuticle.
- At the time of tooth eruption fusion of reduced enamel epithelium with the oral epithelium takes place. The cells in the centre of this fused epithelia degenerate due to lack of nutrition and thus a perforation is formed which creates a passage for the crown to emerge into the oral cavity. The REE remains attached to the portion of enamel that has not yet erupted.
- As tooth eruption progresses, the REE progressively diminishes, resulting in the formation of a shallow groove known as the gingival sulcus between the gingiva and the tooth surface. This groove surrounds the entire tooth.
- But a small portion of REE is still attached on the tooth surface and it forms the junctional epithelium.

****

Q16) Mucogingival junction.

Answer – It is a junction between the gingiva and alveolar mucosa.

- Clinically, it is recognized as the connection between bright pink alveolar mucosa and pale pink gingiva. This juncture is histologically characterized by a slight depression known as the *mucogingival groove*.
- On the palate this junction cannot be recognized as it lacks sharpness. This junction is visible on the mandible's lingual surface as a boundary between the mucosa of the floor of mouth and the gingiva.
- This junction lies approximately 3–5 mm below the alveolar bone's crest.
- Histologically, this junction can be distinguished by the variations in the gingival and oral mucosal epithelium and lamina propria. In lamina propria of gingiva, coarse collagen fiber bundles are attached directly to the periosteum covering the bone and it also possesses a thin keratinized epithelium. There is no submucosal layer. The epithelial rete ridges of gingiva are slender, long and numerous. Whereas the epithelium of alveolar mucosa is thick and nonkeratinized. Its epithelial rete ridges here are short and few. Its lamina propria has numerous small blood vessels close to the surface which gives it a bright pink colour. Submucosa layer is present.

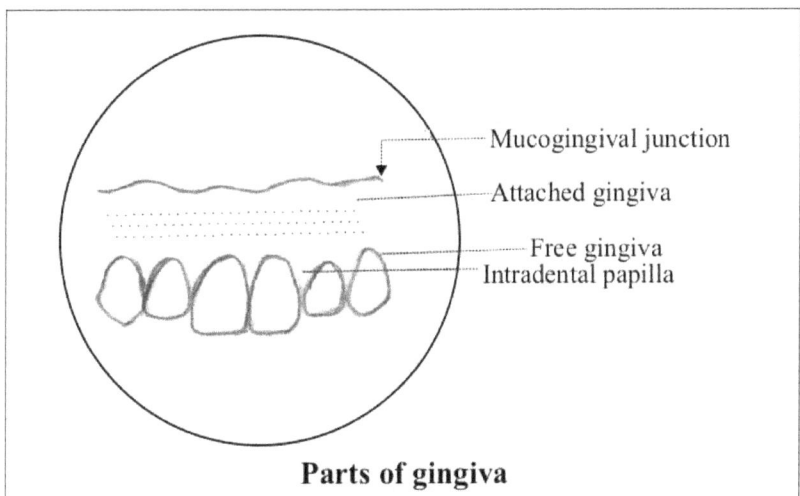

Parts of gingiva

****

Q17) Functions of oral mucosa.

Answer – The moist lining of the oral cavity connecting to the external environment is known as the "oral mucous membrane" or "oral mucosa."

Oral mucosa performs many functions as follows.....

Protection: The oral mucous membrane acts as a barrier, safeguarding the underlying tissues and organs from mechanical damage inflicted by food particles and chewing forces.

Defense: Oralmucosa is not penetrable by bacterial toxins. Additionally, it secretes antibodies, which results in effective immunity.

Sensation: The oral mucosa is responsive to pressure, temperature (both hot and cold), tactile stimuli and sense of smell. Taste perception occurs in the first two-thirds of the dorsum of tongue. Mucosal receptors trigger the responses of swallowing, gagging, and salivating.

Lubrication: Saliva secreted by tiny salivary glands in the oral mucosa keeps it moist and prevents it from drying out and cracking. Moistness also helps in talking, perception of taste, deglutition and mastication.

****

Q18) Basement membrane and basal lamina.

Answer – Connective tissue and epithelium are closely related. At the junction of connective tissue and epithelium, two distinct structures are seen.

a) *Basement membrane* – It is seen at light microscopic level.

b) *Basal lamina* – It is seen at electron microscopic level.

Basement membrane

▶ The basement membrane is the dense barrier between epithelium and connective tissue observable at the light microscope level.

▶ It is relatively cell-free and consists of reticular fibers.

Basal lamina

➢ Under electron microscope, basement membrane is called basal lamina.

➢ At the intersection of the epithelium and CT, it appears as a bright, structure less band in sections stained with periodic acid-Schiff.

➢ *It is made up of two zones.*

1) *Lamina lucida* – A distinct area observed just beneath the epithelial cells.

2) *Lamina densa* – A dark area adjacent to the connective tissue and beneath the lamina lucida. Loops are created in the lamina densa by anchoring fibrils, which are type VII collagen. Collagen types I and II pass into these loops created by type VII collagen. In the lamina densa, type IV collagen also creates a net-like pattern.

****

Q19) Lamina propria.

Answer – The connective tissue of various thicknesses that lies beneath the epithelium is called lamina propria.

- It provides support to the overlying epithelium.
- Within the ground material neurons, blood arteries, collagen and elastic fibers, and a variety of cell types, that include fibroblasts, mast cells, macrophages, and inflammatory cells are present.
- Collagen fibers are mainly type I and type III.
- Lamina propria may attach on to the periosteum covering the alveolar bone or may lie on the submucosa, depending upon the region of the mouth.
- Interlocking of epithelial rete ridges and connective tissue papillae increases surface area and helps disperse the forceapplied onto the overlying epithelium over a larger area of the underlying connective tissue. It facilitates connective tissue epithelium-blood vascular material exchange.
- For the purpose of understanding it is divided into two parts, both of which are in continuum and are not separate portions – Papillary portion and reticular portion.

Papillary portion

- It is a superficial layer present in between the epithelial rete ridges.
- It may be absent or very short in some areas e.g. – alveolar mucosa.
- It has numerous capillary loops and thin, loosely organized collagen fibers.

Reticular portion

- Reticular portion is always present below the papillary portion.
- It contains collagen fibers that are in thick bundles.

****

Q20) Differences between keratinized and non keratinized epithelium.

Answer –

Sl. No.	Keratinized	Non keratinized
1.	Cornified surface layer (contains dead cells)	No cornified surface layer (contains living cells)
2.	Four layers	Three layers
3.	Stratum spinosum cells are smaller	Stratum intermedium cells are larger
4.	Intercellular space is distended (hence prickly appearance)	Cells are closely attached (hence no prickly appearance)
5.	Stratum granulosum and corneum layers are present	Absent
6,	Mitosis comparatively less rate	High rate
7.	Epithelium is thinner	It is thicker
8.	Papillae are high and close.	Papillae are short and spaced.

9.	Keratin present on the surface	No keratin
10.	Keratohyaline granules are present.	These granules are absent
11.	Effective barrier	Comparatively less effective barrier
12.	Superficial layer shows no nuclei (or pyknotic nuclei)	Superficial layer shows viable nuclei

****

SALIVARYGLANDS

MAIN QUESTION

Q1) Describe in detail the ductoacinar unit of salivary glands and add a note on composition and functions of saliva.

Answer -- Saliva is secreted by a set of compound exocrine glands called salivary glands. Since their secretions are expelled through ducts, they are known as exocrine glands. Saliva, a complex fluid that maintains the oral cavity wet, is produced and secreted by the salivary glands as their primary function.

STRUCTURE OF TERMINAL SECRETORY UNIT

- Acini, also known as terminal secretory units or secretory end pieces, are the fundamental unit of the salivary gland.
- Each acinus is made up of serous and mucous cells secretory cells. These cells together with myoepithelial cells are arranged in an acinus. It is spherical shape in serous acini and tubular shape in mucous acini and has a central lumen.
- The cells in each acinus are arranged in a single layer on the basement membrane. Junctional complex holds the cells together in the acini.
- The myoepithelial cells are located on the outer layer of the acini.
- The extension of the lumen between the secretory cells in an acinus gives the central lumen a "star"-like appearance. Each acinus's central lumen steadily enlarges and merges with others before joining the main excretory duct.

SEROUS CELLS

- Serous cells are involved in saliva formation, secretion, and storage.
- Terminal secretory end composed of serous cells is spherical in shape and consists of 8-12 pyramidal-shaped serous cells surrounding a central lumen. The apex of serous cells is narrow near the lumen and broad toward the basement membrane.
- Intercellular canaliculi are finger-like projections observed in the lumen in-between adjacent serous cells.
- The base of serous cells has a rounded nucleus. The apical or luminal region of the cytoplasm consists of a large number of secretory granules. The golgi complex and rER are densely packed in the basal cytoplasm.
- The cells in the acini are held together by a variety of junctional complexes that also control permeability.

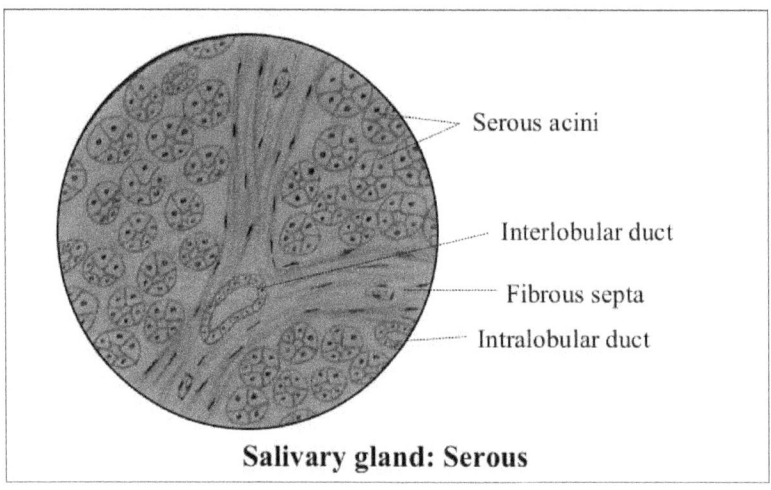
Salivary gland: Serous

MUCOUS CELLS

- Similar to serous cells, mucous cells are also involved in saliva formation, storage and secretion.
- The mucous cell-based terminal secretory end piece is tubular in shape. The end piece appears round with the mucous cells surrounding the lumen when cut in cross sections. Compared to the serous end piece, the lumen is bigger.
- Serous cells form a crescent-shaped coating on the mucous secretory end parts of major and some small salivary glands (serous demilunes). A junctional complex joins the mucous and serous cells.
- The serous cells present in the demilunes are comparable to those in the serous end pieces. Their secretions passes through the intercellular canaliculi that run between the mucous cells to reach the central lumen located in the middle of the secretory end piece.
- Mucous cells are characterized by a significant amount of their secretory product, (mucous) in the basal cytoplasm, which forces the nucleus up against the basal membrane of the cell. The nucleus appears flat as a result. At the base of the compressed cytoplasm are rER, mitochondria and different cell organelles are present.
- Mucous cells usually do not have intercellular canaliculi as do the serous cells. Only those covered by serous demilunes have intercellular canaliculi.

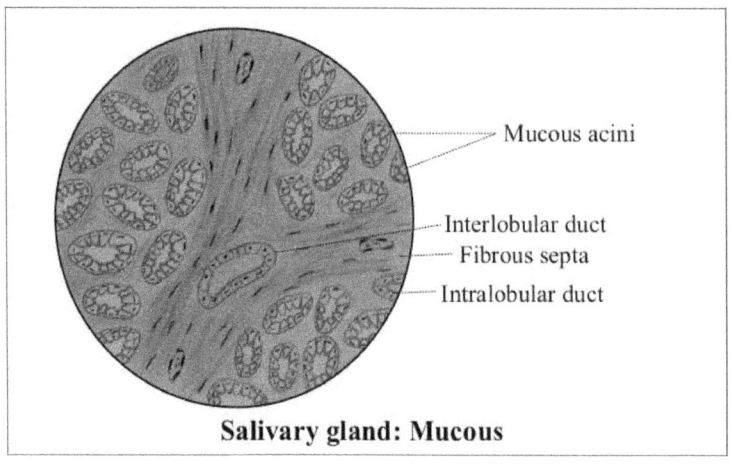
Salivary gland: Mucous

MYOEPITHELIAL CELLS

- Myoepithelial cells, which are contractile cells, are located on the intercalated duct and secretory end piece of the salivary glands.
- Due to their basket-like appearance, they are also called 'basket cells'.
- They are attached to the secretory or ductal cells by desmosomes and are located between them and the basal lamina.
- Their bodies exhibit a stellate morphology, characterized by a flattened nucleus, little cytoplasm and numerous branching processes that surround and envelop the secretory end segment.
- The myoepithelial cells have cytokeratin intermediate filament, actin and myosin which have contractile functions.

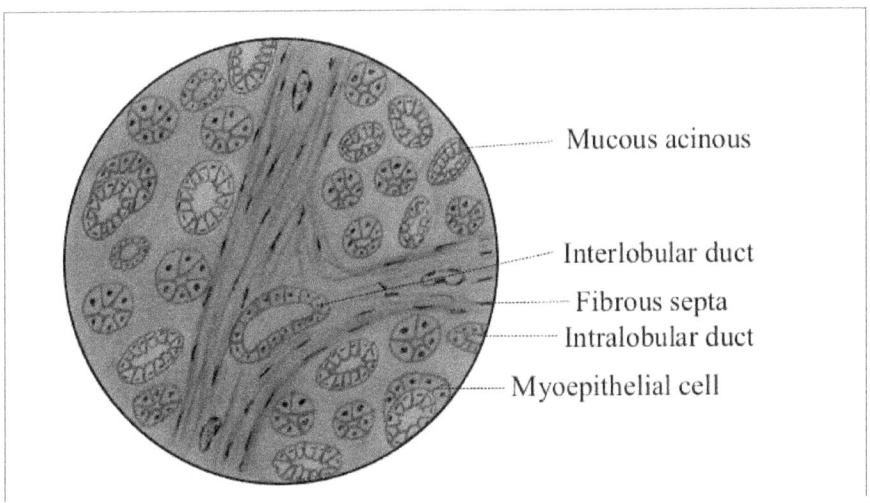

DUCTS

- The ductal system of the salivary glands, extending from the secretory end piece to the oral cavity, has a network of hollow tubules that progressively increase in width.
- The ductal system is not just a simple pipeline for the passage of the saliva. These ducts also participate in the production and modification of saliva.
- The structure and function of the 3 various kinds of ducts -- excretory, striated and intercalated varies. The tiniest duct is the intercalated duct. It connects the terminal secretory units to the succeeding larger duct i.e., striated duct. These smaller ducts join to each other and get larger until main excretory duct is created.
- The location of the ductal system determines its naming. *Intralobular ducts* are the ducts found inside lobules. *Interlobular ducts* are those that are found in between the lobules. Intralobular ducts are classified into two types: *striated* and *intercalated*. Interlobular ducts include the *excretory ducts*.

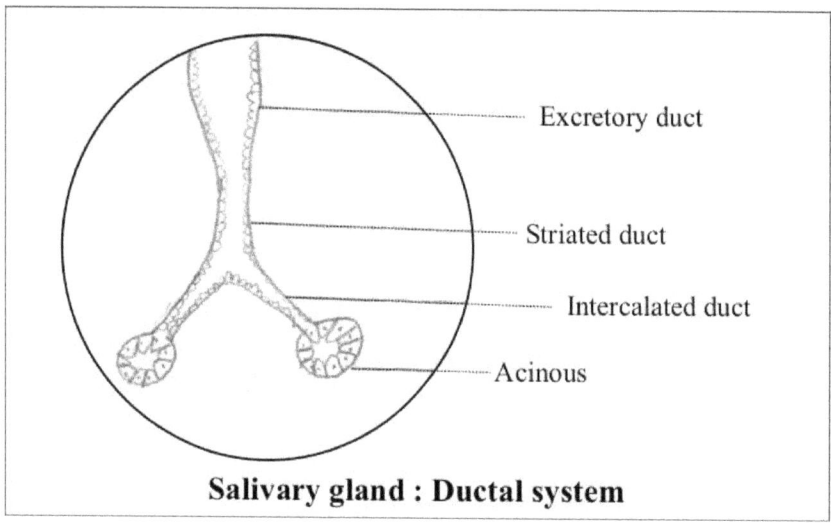

Salivary gland : Ductal system

Intercalated ducts

- Intercalated ducts are intralobular ducts and smallest of all ducts.
- It is the duct in which the primary saliva produced in secretary end piece passes first.
- A single layer of cuboidal cells lines these channels. They possess minimal number of cell organelles and a circular nucleus in the middle.
- The lumen of intercalated duct and secretary end piece are continuous.
- *Functions* – Passage and modification of saliva through secretary and absorptive process. They add macromolecular components like lysozymes and lactoferrin. They have undifferentiated cells that can develop to replace cells that are dead or damaged.

Striated ducts

- Primary saliva from the intercalated ducts is passed on to the next larger duct i.e. striated duct.
- The intralobular ductal system's largest ducts are striated ducts.
- Tall columnar cells with a large, round nucleus positioned in their center line these ducts.

  Functions – By secreting potassium and bicarbonate and reabsorbing sodium and chloride, it changes primary saliva composition. It converts slightly hypertonic or isotonic saliva into hypotonic. It also modifies the organic content of the primary saliva. Ductal cells also synthesize and secrete glycoproteins. Proteins from the luminal surface are reabsorbed by striated ducts.

Excretory ducts

- A lobule's striated ducts combine to generate greater intralobular ducts. These ducts progressively enlarge to form the next largest excretory duct.
- Excretory ducts are found in the connective tissue septa that run between the gland's lobules.
- It is the largest duct, lined with pseudostratified columnar epithelial cells. It transitions to stratified squamous epithelium at the point of merger with the epithelium of the mouth.
- Collagen along with elastic fibers in the CT surrounding the excretory duct allows passive stretching of the duct for accommodation and passage of varying amounts of saliva.

- Excretory ducts play no role in modification of saliva.

'Composition and functions of saliva' refer main question Q2 in chapter "Salivary glands".

****

Q2) Composition, formation, and functions of saliva.

Answer–

COMPOSITION OF SALIVA

- Saliva contains predominantly mainly water (99% or more), with minimal quantities of inorganic ions, glycoproteins, secretory proteins, and different compounds (1% or less).

Electrolytes	Na^+, K^+, Ca^{2+}, Cl^-, HCO^3, HPO^2_4.
Secretory proteins	Amylase, ribonuclease, lysozymes, kallikrein, esterase, nystatin, cystatin, lactoferrin, peroxidase, and acid phosphatase are examples of enzymes.
Immunoglobulins	I_gG, I_gM, I_gA.
Small organic substances	Glucose, blood clotting factors, lipid molecules, amino acids, uric acid, urea, hormones.
Other components	Serum albumin, cyclic adenosine monophosphate-binding proteins, insulin, and epidermal growth factor.
Mixed saliva (whole saliva) comprises produced saliva, desquamated oral epithelial cells, bacteria and their byproducts, leukocytes, food detritus, and crevicular fluid.	

FORMATION AND SECRETION OF SALIVA

- There are two stages in the formation of saliva.
- *First stage*– Primary saliva, an isotonic fluid rich in organic substances and water, is generated at this stage by the cells of the intercalated ducts and secretory ends pieces.
- *Second stage* – As the primary saliva passes through the ducts, it undergoes modifications throughout this stage. Electrolyte reabsorption and secretion occur. The saliva is hypotonic when it eventually enters the oral cavity.
- The apical cytoplasm of the secretory end piece cells contains secretory granules produced by the golgi apparatus and rER. The membranes of these granules merge with the cell membrane at luminal surface under appropriate stimulation, facilitating exocytosis to release the contents into the lumen.
- Ca^{2+} is released from intracellular storage by specific enzymes. Cl^- channels in apical cell membrane and K^+ channels in the basolateral cell membrane are opened due to this increase in Ca^{2+} concentration. Due to the opening of the channels, there is movement of Cl^- from the cell into the lumen. To balance the electrochemical gradient, extracellular Na+ is drawn into the

lumen. Because of the elevation in concentration of Na^+ and Cl^- ions in the lumen, water is absorbed through the cells into the lumen to balance the osmotic variation.

FUNCTIONS OF SALIVA

1) **PROTECTION**
   - Saliva keeps the oral tissues from drying out and causing mucosal atrophy and degeneration.
   - It flushes out food debris and nonadherent bacteria. Clearance of sugar will reduce its availability to caries-causing bacteria.
   - Lubrication from mucins and glycoproteins keeps the oral tissues from adhering to one another, there by permitting free movements during mastication and speech.
   - By buffering the temperature and reducing chemical concentrations, saliva protects the oral mucosa from thermal and chemical impacts.
   - Some high molecular weight glycoproteins in saliva aggregate specific strains of oral microbes and there by prevent its binding to the oral tissue and thus facilitate its clearance.

2) **DIGESTION**
   - Saliva increases the solubility of food particles and thus helps in digestion.
   - Salivary enzyme amylase acts on ingested carbohydrates in the food to produce glucose and maltose. Triglycerides are digested into monoglycerides, diglycerides and fatty acids by the enzyme lipase present in saliva.

3) **BUFFERING**
   - Saliva's bicarbonates and phosphate ions operate as a buffer, preventing the teeth from becoming demineralized due to bacteria generated acids.
   - Urea and ammonia, both effective in elevating pH, are generated when bacteria decompose the proteins and peptides present in saliva.

4) **MAINTAINANCE OF TOOTH INTERGRITY**
   - Calcium and phosphate ions are supersaturated in saliva. The tooth's surface hardness and resistance to demineralization are increased when these ions are present in high concentrations.
   - Helps in the early caries remineralization.

5) **ANTIMICROBIAL ACTIVITY**
   - Saliva contains proteins with antibacterial properties, including lysozyme, lactoferrin, and peroxidase.
   - Certain germs are agglutinated by immunoglobulin IgA, which prevents them from adhering to the oral tissues.

6) **TISSUE REPAIR**
   - In experimental settings, salivary peptides and proteins stimulate tissue development, differentiation and wound healing.

7) TASTE PERCEPTION

- Food is solubilized by saliva so that taste receptors in taste buds can detect it.
- Salivary proteins in saliva generated by the small salivary glands located near the vallate papillae have been suggested to bind to the taste compounds and present them to the taste receptors.

8) MASTICATION AND DEGLUTITION

- Food is moistened by saliva. It helps in starting the digestive process by breaking the food down into smaller pieces.
- The lubricating and moisturizing properties of saliva assist deglutition and permit the formation of bolus.
- Saliva reduces temperature of hot foods.

9) SPEECH

- Salivary lubricates oral tissue and keeps it moist. This helps in speech.

****

Q3) Classify salivary glands. Discuss in detail the histology of submandibular salivary gland. Add a note on ductal systems in major salivary glands.

Q) Classify salivary glands. Discuss in detail the histology of mixed salivary glands.

Answer –

CLASSIFICATION OF SALIVARY GLANDS

Based on the size

Major

-Parotid gland

-Submandibular gland

-Sublingual gland

Minor

-Labial and buccal glands

-Glossopalatine glands

-Palatine glands

-Lingual glands (glands of Blandin and Nuhn)

-Von Ebner's glands

Based on the location

-Labial salivary glands

-Lingual salivary glands

Based on the type of secretion

- Serous salivary gland
- Mucous salivary gland
- Mixed salivary gland

SUBMANDIBULAR GLAND

- ***Synonym*** – Submaxillary gland
- The second-largest salivary gland is the submandibular gland.
- It is a mixed salivary gland.
- ***Macroscopy*** -- The gland is situated directly medial to mandibular body in the submandibular triangle. It is located posteriorly and superficially to the mylohyoid muscle, featuring a folded extension at the muscle's posterior border. Wharton's duct serves as the principal excretory duct of submandibular gland. It advances anteriorly over the mylohyoid muscle and positions itself immediately below the mucosa. It opens at the sublingual papillae, also known as the carunculasublingualis, located just lateral to the lingual frenum.
- ***Histology*** – Being a mixed gland it has both serous and mucous secretory units. Although the proportion of serous and mucous end pieces varies from one lobule to the other, serous cells predominates the mucous cells.
- Write about 'serous cells', 'mucous cells', 'myoepithelial cells', and 'duct' from main question Q1 from chapter 'Salivary glands'.

****

Q4) Classify salivary glands and ducts. Explain histology of serous salivary gland.

Q) Classify salivary glands. Explain histology of parotid gland.

Answer– Refer to section 'Classification of salivary glands' in main question Q3 in chapter 'Salivary glands'.

STRUCTURE OF TERMINAL SECRETORY UNIT

- Parotid gland is exclusively a serous gland.
- Refer to sections 'Structure of terminal secretory unit', 'Serous cells', 'Myoepithelial cells', 'Ducts' in main question Q1 in chapter 'Salivary glands'.

Connective tissue (CT)

- The connective tissue of the parotid gland includes a capsule that encloses the gland.
- The gland's lobes and lobules are separated by the extension of the CT of the capsule (called as septa) within the gland. Nerves along with blood arteries that supply the ducts and secretory units are carried by the septa.

- It comprises fibroblasts, plasma cells, macrophages, mast cells, dendritic cells, and adipose tissue, similar to connective tissue located in other regions of the body.

****

SHORT NOTES

Q1) Mucous cell.

Answer -- Refer to section 'Mucous cell' in main question Q1 in chapter 'Salivary glands'.

****

Q2) Serous acini.

Answer -- Refer to section 'Serous cells' in main question Q1 in 'Salivaryglands'.

****

Q3) Difference between mucous and serous glands.

Answer --

DIFFERENCES BETWEEN MUCOUS AND SEROUS CELLS

Sl. No.	Mucous cell	Serous cell
1	*Cell shape* – Pyramidal	Pyramidal but with narrow apex near the lumen.
2	*Nucleus* – It is flat and at the base.	*Nucleus* – It is round at the basal one-third.
3	Apical portion of the cell appears empty.	Apical portion contains zymogen granules.
4	Apical portion stains weakly with H and E.	Apical portion stains strongly with H and E.
5	*Terminal secretory end piece shape* – Elliptical.	Spherical.
6	*Acini size* – Larger.	Smaller.
7	*Lumen size* – Large	Small
8	Intercellular canaliculi are absent.	Intercellular canaliculi are present.
9	Produce more carbohydrate components than proteins.	Produce fewer carbohydrate components than proteins.
10	Secretory droplets are irregular and large.	Secretory droplets are smaller and covered by membrane.
11	Secretion has no enzymatic activity.	Secretion shows enzymatic activity.
12	Golgi complex is located between nucleus and secretory droplets.	Golgi bodies are located apical to the nucleus.

Q4) Demilunes.

Answer -- Serous cells form a crescent-shaped covering over the mucous end pieces of major and some small salivary glands (*serous demilunes*)**.** Serous cells in the demilunes are similar to the serous cells found in serous secretory end piece. The serous and mucous cells are interconnected by a junctional complex. Secretions from the demilunes reach the central lumen of the secretory end piece through the intercellular canaliculi present between the cells.

****

Q5) Saliva

Answer– Refer to main question Q2 in chapter 'Salivaryglands'.

****

Q6) Striated duct.

Answer– Refer to section 'striated duct' in main question Q1 in chapter 'Salivary glands'.

****

Q7) Intercalated duct.

Answer–Refer to section 'intercalated duct' in main question Q1 in chapter 'Salivary glands'.

****

Q8) Myoepithelial cell.

Answer –Refer to section 'Myoepithelial cell' in main question Q1 in chapter 'Salivary glands'.

Functions

- Contraction of the myoepithelial cell provides support to the secretory end piece during active saliva secretion, there by reducing back permeation of the fluid into the secretory cells.
- The pressure developed during contraction helps to expel primary saliva from the secretory end piece into the duct.
- In order to maintain the intercalated ducts clear, the myoepithelial cells on them contract, expanding the channels.
- By generating a variety of proteins with tumor suppressors, these cells operate as a barrier against epithelial malignancies.

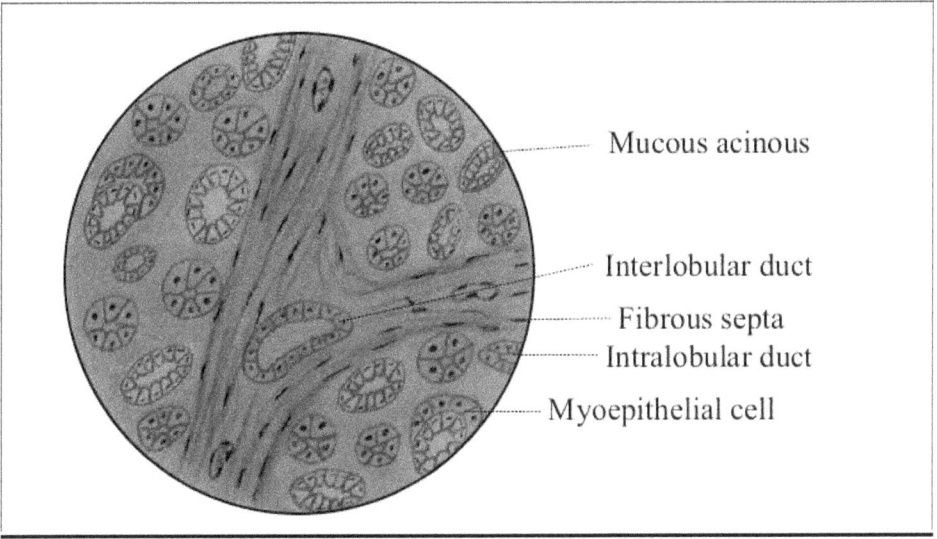

***

Q9) Histology of minor salivary glands.

Answer --

- Almost every area of the oral cavity has many small salivary glands situated beneath the epithelium. The number varies in the oropharynx and oral cavity.
- Aggregates of secretory end pieces and ducts, arranged in tiny lobules in the submucosa or in between tongue muscle fibers, make up minor salivary glands. They don't have a distinct capsule. Individual aggregate ducts open directly onto the mucosal surface.
- They are not present in the gingiva, anterior region of the hard palate and in anterior two thirds of the dorsum of the tongue.

Classification

Location determines the classification of minor salivary glands.

a) Labial glands
b) Buccal glands
c) Lingual glands
d) Palatine glands
e) Glossopalatine glands

Labial and buccal glands

- Minor salivary glands of lip and cheek are mixed type having both mucous secretory end piece and serous demilunes.

Lingual glands

- The tongue's glands can be categorized into many groups.
- *Anterior lingual glands (glands of Blandin and Nuhn)* -- These mucous glands are situated close to the tongue's apex. Their ducts open near the frenum on the tongue's ventral surface.
- *Posterior lingual mucous glands* – these minor glands lie close to the lingual tonsil, and are located lateral and posterior to the circumvallate papillae. Ducts open on the dorsal surface.
- *Posterior lingual serous glands (von Ebner's glands)* –These are pure serous glands situated beneath the circumvallate papilla, between the tongue's muscle fibers. Their ducts open into the circumvallate papilla's trough. The secretions from this gland wash the trough of the vallate papilla so as to keep the taste receptors clean. Apart from this they play a vital role in protective and digestive functions. They produce antibacterial enzymes peroxidase and lysosome and a secretory enzyme with lipolytic activity.

Glossopalatine glands

- They are exclusively mucus glands. They are located in the isthumus region within the glossopalatine fold.

Palatine glands

- The submucosa of the soft palate and uvula, as well as the lamina propria of posterolateral area of the hard palate, contains these pure mucous glands. Their ducts open on the palatal mucosa.

****

TEMPOROMANDIBULAR JOINT

SHORT NOTES

Q1) Anatomy and histology of temporomandibular joint.

Answer – The temporomandibular joint is a condylar-type synovial joint.

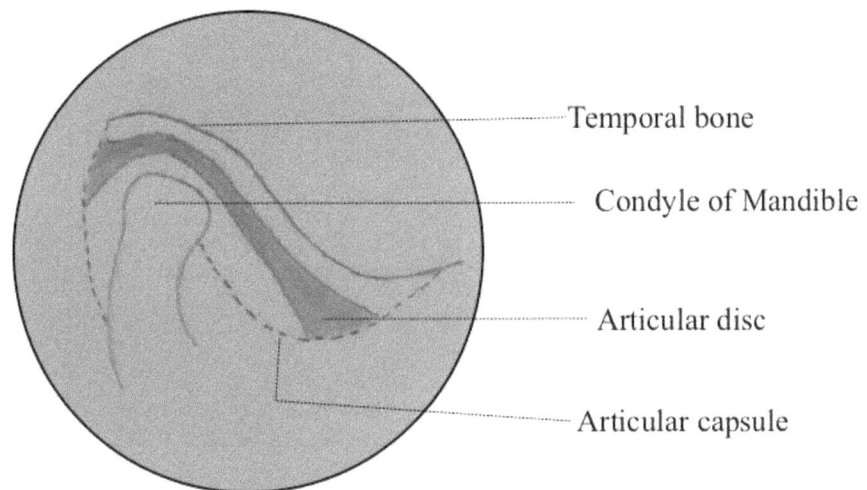

Temporomandibular joint

GROSS ANATOMY

Articular bony structures

- Parts of the temporal bone (the anterior part of the mandibular fossa and the articular tubercle) constitute the upper articular surface.
- The mandibular condylar head forms the lower articular surface.
- The perichondrium covers the articular surfaces.

Condyle of the mandible

- Condyle is convex and oval in shape.
- It is wider lateromedially and anteroposteriorly.
- Its long axis is oriented posteromedially.

Articular disc

- A fibrous disk called an articular disc is interposed between the upper and lower articulating surfaces.
- The disk is oval in shape, fibrous, avascular and noninnervated.

- It is firmly attached to the medial and lateral collateral ligaments.
- It has a concave inferior surface and a concavo-convex superior surface in the sagittal section. Its anterior and posterior bands are thick, whereas its middle zone is thin.

  The disk divides the joint space into two compartments....

  1] <u>Lower compartment (condylodiskal)</u> – It is between the condyle and the disk. It helps in opening the jaws.

  2] <u>Upper compartment (temperodiskal)</u> -- It is between the disk and the temporal bone. It helps in inferior movement of the mandible.

Articular capsule

- "Articular capsule" refers to the fibrous tissue that covers the condyle and articular eminence.
- This fibrous covering is of even thickness in the mandibular condyle.
- The fibrous coating of the temporal bone's articulating surface is thick on the articular eminence's posterior slope and thin in the articular fossa.

Ligaments

- Refer to short notes Q4 in chapter "Temporomandibular joint".

Articular fossa

- The articular fossa (also called mandibular fossa) is a depression on the temporal bone where the condylar head articulates to allow jaw movements.
- It consists of anterior and posterior parts. Anterior part forms the prominence and the posterior part forms depression.
- It is located in front of the auditory canal.

Synovial fluid

- Rich capillary network present in the joint produce the clear, straw-colored fluid known as synovial fluid. It is present in joint spaces.
- It is viscous in nature and its amount decreases with age.

HISTOLOGY

Articular bony structures

- The mandibular condyle is formed of inner cancellous bone and an outer plate of compact bone.
- Large marrow spaces in the cancellous bone contain bony trabeculae. These trabculae radiate from the neck of mandible and reach the cortex at right angles. The marrow space consists of red

bone marrow the quantity of which decreases with age due to progressive thickening of the trabeculae. Red marrow is replaced by fatty or yellow marrow with ageing.

- A thin layer of compact bone makes up the glenoid fossa.
- Articular eminence is made of compact bone having an inner core of cancellous bone.

Articular disk

- The articular disk of younger individuals is made up of thick, fibrous connective tissue.
- In young, the fibroblasts are elongated, spindle shaped having thing long processes. With ageing, they appear rounded and are arranged in pairs similar to chondroid cells.

Articular capsule

- It is thick fibroelastic tissue made up of strong collagenous fibers.
- It contains fibroblasts and few chondrocytes. Chondrocytes number increase with ageing.
- The fibrous tissue is arranged in two layers -- inner fibrous zone and outer fibrous zone, with a small transitional zone in between. The collagen fibers in the inner zone are orientated perpendicularly to the bony surface, while in the outer zone, they are aligned parallelly.
- Variable numbers of chondrocytes are found on the temporal surface.

****

Q2) Articular capsule.

Answer –

Gross anatomy

- The fibrous tissue casing the articular eminence and condyle is referred to as the articular capsule.
- While the fibrous covering on the temporal bone is dense on the posterior slope of the articular eminence and thin in the articular fossa. It is uniformly thick in the mandibular condyle.
- It is devoid of nerves and blood vessels and thus has limited reparative capacity.

Histology

- It is thick fibroelastic tissue made up of strong collagen fibers.
- It contains fibroblasts and few chondrocytes. Chondrocytes number increase with aging.
- The fibrous tissue is organized into two layers: an inner fibrous zone and an outer fibrous zone, separated by a minor transitional zone. The collagen fibers are parallel to the bony surface in the outer zone and at right angles to it in the inner zone.

****

Q3) Articular disc of TMJ.

Answer– Articular disc is a fibrous disk that is interposed in between the articulating surfaces of TMJ.

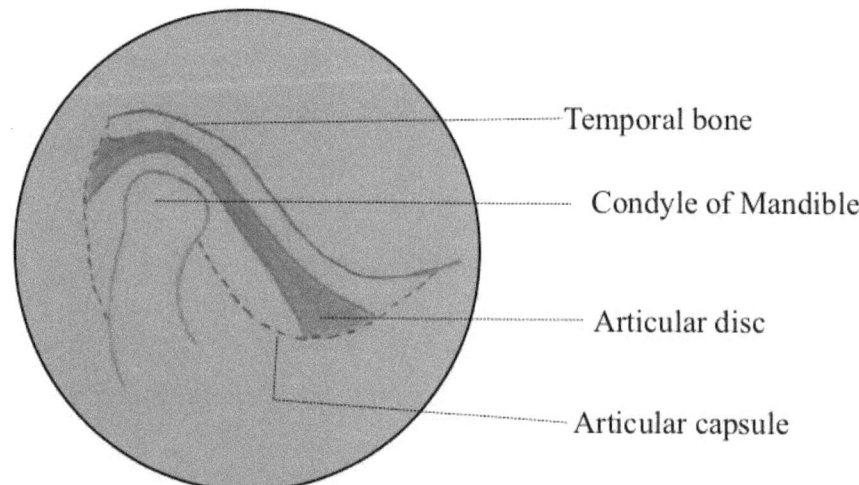

Temporomandibular joint

Gross anatomy

- The disk is oval in shape, fibrous, avascular, and noninnervated.
- Both the medial and lateral collateral ligaments have a firm attachment to it.
- It has a concave inferior surface and a concavo-convex superior surface in sagittal section. It is characterized by a thin middle zone and dense anterior and posterior bands.

Histology

- In younger individuals, the articular disk has dense fibrous connective tissue.
- In young, the fibroblasts are elongated having thing long processes. With ageing, these appear rounded and arranged in pairs similar to chondroid cells.

Functions

a) It assists in absorption of shock and performs as a cushion.
b) The disc lessens the friction between the articulating surfaces.
c) It allows condylar movement during gliding.
d) It fills the space between the articulating surfaces, thereby stabilizing the condyle.

The disk divides the joint space into two compartments....

1] <u>Lower compartment (condylodiskal)</u> – It is between the condyle and the disk. It helps in opening the jaws.

2] <u>Upper compartment (temperodiskal)</u> -- It is between the disk and the temporal bone. It facilitates the inferior movement of the mandible.

****

Q4) Enumerate the ligaments of temporomandibular joint and their functions.

<u>Answer</u> – The temporomandibular joint comprises the following ligaments……

a) ***Lateral temporomandibular ligament*** – It runs obliquely downward and backward from the articular eminence lateral aspect to the condylar neck's posterior aspect. *Functions* – i) serves as the primary support for the joint; ii) prevents joint dislocation by restricting the distal and inferior movements of the mandible.

b) ***Sphenomandibular ligament*** –It is an additional ligament traversing between the lingula positioned near the mandibular foramen and the spine of the sphenoid bone. *Functions* -- It limits the inferior distension of the mandible.

c) ***Stylomandibular ligament*** – This ligament is attached above to the lateral surface of the styloid process and below to the angle of the mandible. *Functions* -- It limits the excessive protrusive movements of the mandible.

****

Q5) Bony structures of TMJ.

<u>Answer</u> -- Temporomandibular joint is a synovial joint of condylar type.

GROSS ANATOMY

- Parts of the temporal bone (the anterior part of the mandibular fossa and the articular tubercle) constitute the upper articular surface.
- The mandibular condylar head forms the lower articular surface.
- The perichondrium covers the articular surfaces.

<u>Condyle of the mandible</u>

- Condyle is convex and oval in shape.
- It is wider lateromedially and anteroposteriorly.
- Its long axis is oriented posteromedially.

HISTOLOGY

- The mandibular condyle is formed of inner cancellous bone and an outer plate of compact bone.
- Large marrow spaces in the cancellous bone contain bony trabeculae. These trabeculae radiate from the neck of mandible and reach the cortex at right angles. The marrow space consists of red

bone marrow the quantity of which decreases with age due to progressive thickening of the trabeculae. Red marrow is replaced by fatty or yellow marrow with ageing.

- A thin layer of compact bone makes up the glenoid fossa.
- Articular eminence is made of compact bone having an inner core of cancellous bone.

****

TOOTH ERUPTION AND SHEDDING

MAIN QUESTIONS

Q1) Describe in detail the mechanism of tooth eruption.

Answer–

- "Eruption" is the Latin word "erumpere" meaning to breakout.
- **_Definition_** -- Eruption is the word employed to describe the transition of a tooth from its developmental position in the jaw to its functional position in the occlusal plane.

Physiologic phases of tooth movement

There are three physiologic phases of tooth movement....

a) Pre eruptive tooth movement.
b) Eruptive tooth movement.
c) Post eruptive tooth movement.

Pre-eruptive tooth movement

- These movements are made by a tooth germ within the osseous crypt of the jaw prior to eruption.
- When deciduous tooth germ forms, they are small and have a good space between them. Due to the rapid growth of the tooth germs, crowding occurs. Growth of jaw will relieve this crowding by the movement of the tooth germs. Bone remodeling of the crypt wall will allow further movement of the growing tooth germs.
- Pre-eruptive tooth movements within the bony crypt are also observed in permanent teeth, regardless of whether they have deciduous predecessors.

Histology

- Pre-eruptive tooth movement in the form of growth of tooth germs or its movements to relieve crowding requires bony wall remodeling. The selective resorption and deposition of bone by osteoclasts and osteoblasts respectively, achieve this purpose (bone remodeling).

Eruptive tooth movement

- The movement a tooth undergoes from its initial location in the jaw to its final functional position in the occlusal plane is termed as eruptive tooth movements.
- The main movement of the tooth germ is towards the occlusal direction.
- Once the tooth just erupts into the oral cavity, the movements made by it to reach the occlusal plane is termed as 'pre-functional' eruptive tooth movements.

Histology

- In this phase of tooth movement, various histological changes emerge, like the development of periodontal ligament, dentogingival junction and roots.
- Root development is initiated by HERS. It prompts the odontoblast differentiation from dental papilla cells. The odontoblasts subsequently secrete root dentin, there by elongating the root length.
- Cementum, periodontal ligament and the bone that lines the cavity wall are formed shortly after the first stage of root formation.
- Numerous structural changes are also seen in the pdl which could favor the tooth movement. Fibroblasts in periodontal ligament have dual functions and are responsible for simultaneous synthesis along with degradation of collagen fibers.
- Significant histological changes also occur in the tissue overlying the erupting tooth. Removal of the overlying bone is necessary for the permanent tooth to erupt. When the deciduous teeth erupt, the permanent tooth which is apically located is completely surrounded by bone except for a small canal filled with connective tissue containing remnants of dental lamina (gubernacular cord). This cord may guide the permanent tooth as it erupts.
- The fusion of the oral epithelium and reduced enamel epithelium takes place. The cells in the centre of this fused epithelia degenerate due to lack of nutrition and thus a perforation is created which allows easy passage for the crown to emerge into the oral cavity.

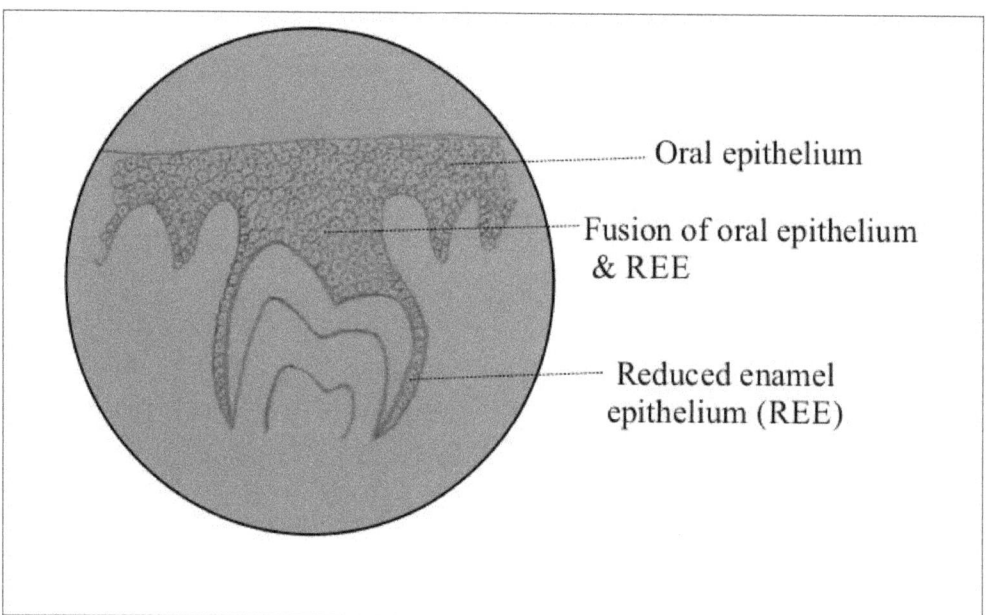

Post-eruptive tooth movement.

    a) After attaining its final functional position in occlusion, certain movements are performed by a tooth which is known as post-eruptive tooth movements. It is of two types.

a) *Movements that maintain the position of the erupted tooth even when the jaw growth is taking place* -- The movement is mainly in the occlusal direction to maintain pace with the increasing height of the jaws. It involves both the tooth and its socket and stops when the jaw growth is completed.
b) *Movements that compensate for the occlusal and the proximal wear* -- These movements occur throughout life and involve occlusal and mesial migration of the tooth. Proximal wear decreases the arch length which is compensated by the mesial drifting of the tooth.

Histology

- Histologically, during the post-eruptive phase, the position of the tooth socket is adjusted through the production of new bone at the alveolar crest and the socket floor.
- Continued cementum deposition at the root apex may compensate for occlusal wear. Osteoclasts and osteoblasts cause the mesial drifting of teeth by resorbing bone on mesial side and depositing bone on the distal side of the socket wall respectively.

****

Q2) Enumerate and describe theories of eruption of teeth.

Answer –

- **Definition** -- Eruption is the word employed to describe the transition of a tooth from its developmental position in the jaw to its functional position in the occlusal plane.
- The movement of tooth during eruption is impacted by a number of different factors.
- *Mechanism of tooth eruption although not completely clear, few theories have been proposed to explain it.*
   a) Bone remodeling theory.
   b) Root elongation theory (cushion hammock ligament theory).
   c) Vascular pressure theory.
   d) Pulp constriction theory.
   e) Periodontal ligament traction theory.

Bone remodeling theory

- This theory postulates that selective bone growth and resorption in the socket facilitates tooth eruption.
- Bone remodeling is essential for facilitating movements of the tooth.
- Experimentally, the dental follicle was left in place and the tooth germ was extracted. The overlying bone developed an eruptive channel. Similarly, if a silicon or metal replica was replaced for a tooth germ, it also erupted. If the dental follicle was removed, and the tooth germ left intact, then there was no formation of eruptive pathway. These experiments prove that dental follicle is absolutely required for bone remodeling and tooth eruption. Osteoblasts and osteoclasts whose functions are bone deposition and removal respectively are produced in the dental follicle.

Root elongation theory (cushion hammock ligament theory)

- This concept suggests that occlusal movement occurs when a developing root exerts pressure on a stationary structure, thereby utilizing this apically directed force in occlusal movement.
- Few suggested that a band of fibrous tissue (cushion hammock ligament) exists below the root apex running from one side to the other of the alveolar socket wall. Tooth eruption occurs when the tooth applies pressure on this ligament (similar to bow and arrow).
- But when clinically, experimentally and histologically interpreted, results go against this theory. When a tooth that is about to erupt is fixed to the surrounding bone, root growth and bone resorption at the base of the socket continued. But histologically no fixed structure was noted at the base of the socket.
- Clinical observations show that eruptive tooth movement is not caused by root lengthening. For instance, some teeth shift farther distance compared to their root length. Teeth that have no roots also erupted.

Vascular pressure theory

- According to this concept, a localized rise in vascular pressure at the root's apex can generate enough pressure to cause tooth movement.
- Experiments conducted show hypotensive drugs increase hydrostatic pressure and there by there was increase in the rate of eruption. Similarly sympathetic nerve stimulation causes vasoconstriction, thereby decreasing the hydrostatic pressure and reducing the rate of eruption.
- *Evidence* -- Many fenestrated capillaries found at the base of the bony crypt of a tooth which showed greater rate of eruption.
- *Drawback* – i) Only hydrostatic pressure may be insufficient to cause tooth eruption for long periods, ii) tooth eruption was noted even when the vascular supply was cut.

Pulp constriction theory

- According to this theory, the pulp becomes constricted as the root dentin grows, which generates enough pressure to move the tooth occlusally.
- *Drawback* – pulp less teeth also erupt at the same rate as normal teeth.

Periodontal ligament traction theory

- This is the most widely accepted theory.
- It posits that the cells and fibers within the dental follicle and periodontal ligament regulate the movement of teeth into the mouth cavity.
- Presence of eruptive force in the dental follicle and PDL is supported by multiple experiments.
- To provide the requisite force for tooth eruption, periodontal ligament fibroblasts can contract and transmit the contractile force to the collagen fibers. These fibers must remodel and be inclined in appropriate direction to bring about tooth movement. Any disturbances in its remodeling will interfere with eruption.

- Experiments in which the root was cut and a metal barrier placed in between showed the eruption of the distal fragment. This suggests that the fragment erupted because of its attachment to the dental follicle.
- *Drawback* – i) Experiments have shown few teeth having periodontal ligament failed to erupt, ii) even rootless teeth erupted.
- Abnormalities of dental follicles in certain diseases were associated with delay in tooth eruption.
- Drugs inhibiting collagen fiber formation in pdl affected eruption.

****

SHORT NOTES

Q 1) Theories of tooth eruption.

Q2) Enumerate the theories of tooth eruption and write in short about the most accepted one.

Answer – Refer to main question Q2 in chapter "Eruption and shedding"

****

Q3) Periodontal ligament traction theory.

Answer – Refer to section 'Periodontal ligament traction theory' in main question Q2 in chapter "Eruption and shedding"

****

Q4) Pre-eruptive tooth movement.

Answer – "Eruption" is the Latin word 'erumpere' meaning to breakout.

- Eruption is the word employed to describe the transition of a tooth from its developmental position in the jaw to its functional position in the occlusal plane.

Physiologic phases of tooth movement (TM)

There are three physiologic phases of tooth movement...

- ✓ Pre eruptive tooth movement.
- ✓ Eruptive tooth movement.
- ✓ Post eruptive tooth movement.

Refer to section 'Pre-eruptive tooth movement' in main question Q1 in chapter "Eruption and shedding".

****

Q5) Shedding of teeth

Q) Shedding of deciduous teeth.

Answer –

Definition – Exfoliation, also known as shedding, is the physiological process that causes the deciduous teeth to be completely eliminated.

Pattern of shedding

- Shedding occurs as a result of progressive resorption of roots of the deciduous teeth and its supporting tissues.
- The pressure exerted by the growing and erupting permanent teeth directs the pattern of deciduous root resorption.
- *Incisors* -- Permanent tooth germs in mandible are placed more lingual to the deciduous incisor roots. Initially, pressure is applied to the lingual surface of the deciduous tooth, resulting in resorption of root on that side. With continued root resorption, the developing permanent tooth germ occupies a location directly below the deciduous tooth root.
- *Molars* -- Resorption of roots of deciduous molar first begins on the inner surface. This is because the developing premolars are found in between the deciduous roots. When the premolars begin to erupt complete root resorption occurs and the deciduous molar is shed.

Mechanism of resorption and shedding

- The pressure that the erupting permanent teeth exert is a significant factor in shedding since odontoclasts are observable where the pressure is applied. Odontoclasts are large, multinucleated cells that remove dental hard tissue. They occupy resorption bay on the dental surface that is being resorbed.
- Reduced enamel epithelium covering the erupting permanent tooth may release some substances that might initiate the resorption process.
- Monocytes migrate from blood the vessels to the resorption site. They differentiate into odontoclasts which release enzymes and acids which is necessary to break down the dentin and cementum. It adhers to the root surface through a ruffled border. Under electron microscope, this ruffled border is extensive folding of cell membrane.
- Near the ruffled border of odontoclast, there is an area in the cytoplasm where no organelles are present. This clear zone acts as an attachment apparatus for the odontoclast. Cytoplasm of the odontoclast has high concentration of vacuoles containing acid phosphatase adjacent to the ruffled border. Addition of hydrogen ions by the ruffled border in the extracellular compartment further acidifies it so that mineral dissolution occurs. Lysosomes secrete enzymes in the same environment which degrade the organic matrix.

Q6) Histology of shedding.

Answer –

Definition – Shedding or exfoliation is the physiological process that causes the deciduous teeth to be completely eliminated.

Refer to section 'Mechanism of resorption and shedding' in short notes Q5 in chapter "Eruption and shedding"

****

Bibiography

1) Orban's Oral Histology, Embryology and Physiology. G. S. Kumar. Sixteenth edition. Elsevier.

2) Wheelers Dental Anatomy, Physiology and Occlusion. Stanley J, Nelson. Eleventh edition. Elsevier.

3) Manual of Oral Histology and Oral Pathology. Color Atlas and Text. Maji Jose. Third edition. CBS publishers & Distributors Pvt Ltd.

4) Concise Medical Physiology. Sujeet K. Chaudhuri. Sixth edition. New Central Book agency (P) Ltd.

5) Human Anatomy. B D Chaurasia. Volume 3. Sixth edition. CBS publishers & Distributors Pvt Ltd.

www.ingramcontent.com/pod-product-compliance
Lightning Source LLC
LaVergne TN
LVHW070603070526
838199LV00011B/473